MW01041880

"Every month there are about ten new 'guaranteed to work' miracle diets, which yields about 120 per year. Since this has been going for years, there have been hundreds of such diets. If even one had succeeded in maintaining the initial weight loss, wouldn't it have survived?

Instead of adding another new diet, Dr. Schwartz has come up with a program that focuses on eating as a spiritual experience. ***Holy Eating*** is a unique approach that involves an overall shift towards a more spiritual life. Taken seriously, this method can yield not only sustained weight control, but also a happier and more purposeful life."

Rabbi Abraham Twerski, M.D.
Founder & Medical Director Emeritus
Gateway Rehabilitation Center
Internationally renowned psychiatrist and expert on addictions, Dr. Twerski is the author of more than sixty books on spirituality and self-improvement.

"This interesting book adds a new dimension to understanding the principles of healthy eating and will provide motivation for dietary change to those who are open to its message."

Akiva Tatz, M.D.
Author of *Dangerous Disease and Dangerous Therapy in Jewish Medical Ethics* and other works.

In the ***Holy Eating*** program, the focus goes beyond calories and carbs to the individual and his relationship with the physical and the spiritual, the self and the soul. I have experienced weight loss, but even more rewarding is that I have developed a spiritual, holistic relationship with food–and I've enjoyed the process. The primary focus is not on weight *lost*, but on weight *transformed*, from stored energy – in the form of fat – to spent energy, in the form of life."

Paul Herman, M.Ed., LPC
Licensed Professional Counselor, Certified Addiction Counselor

"***Holy Eating*** gives you the tools for optimal emotional, physical and spiritual health, in addition to sustainable weight loss. I trust Dr. Schwartz with my clients because his advice and insights make sense, and they work."

Arden Zinn,
Founder, Arden's Garden Health Food Products

HOLY EATING

◆ ◆ ◆ ◆ ◆ ◆ ◆

The Spiritual Secret to Eternal Weight Loss

ROBERT M. SCHWARTZ, PH.D.

Illustrated by Shoshannah Brombacher, Ph.D.

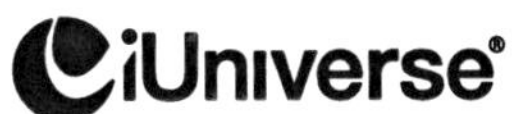

Holy Eating
The Spiritual Secret to Eternal Weight Loss

iUniverse books may be ordered through booksellers or by contacting:

iUniverse
1663 Liberty Drive
Bloomington, IN 47403
www.iuniverse.com
1-800-Authors (1-800-288-4677)

ISBN: 978-1-4620-6344-4 (sc)
ISBN: 978-1-4620-6345-1 (e)

Print information available on the last page.

iUniverse rev. date: 09/04/2015

Scripture quotations are taken from The Artscroll Series––Stone Edition (2003)
Mesorah Publications, Brooklyn, NY

Contents

Part III: How to Make Your Meals Holy

PART IV: NOT A DIET AND HOW TO STAY ON IT

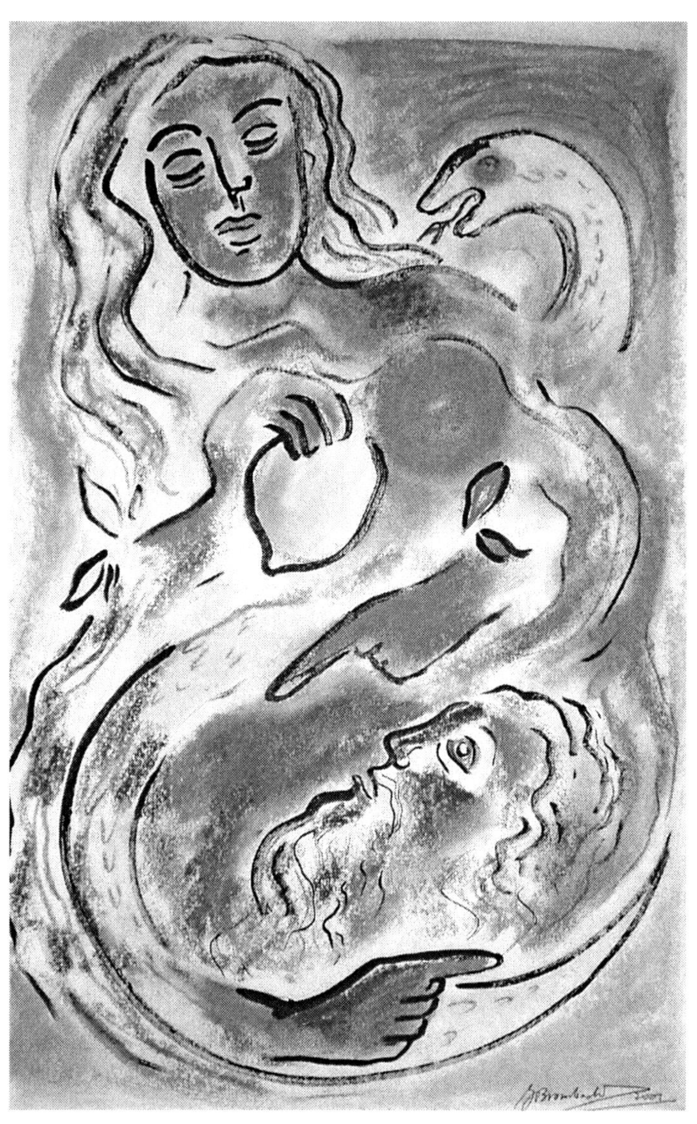

Adam and Eve

Preface: The Journey from Psychology to Spirituality

"God must have loved calories because He made so many of them."
—Anonymous

As I reached the midpoint of my life's journey, I could look back on many successes. With focus and determination, I had been able to overcome many obstacles—with the exception of one. Over the years I gradually bloated up, becoming 50 pounds overweight. I could not maintain weight loss. I am a psychotherapist, so my clients would often ask me to help them lose weight. Although I am an expert in facilitating behavior change, I would tell them frankly:

> "I can help you overcome your depression and anxiety, and teach you self-control strategies. But the research on weight loss shows that even with major medical problems people generally can't lose weight *and maintain the loss.* If they do shed pounds, they gain them back. Only about 5 percent are consistently successful. Furthermore, I myself can't slim down, so how can I help you? When you are feeling better and figure out how to lose weight, please let *me* know!"

In 25 years of practice, no one had taken me up on the challenge. Finally, someone did. Jack's father had lost 50 pounds on the Atkins low carbohydrate diet years before it became the latest craze, when the medical establishment still viewed it as unhealthy. So my client and his wife tried the Atkins diet and both lost about 30 pounds. That's a lot of pounds for one family! I was intrigued and excited. After all these years, one of my clients had taken my quip seriously and actually brought me a weight loss success story.

I read the Atkins diet book voraciously, cut back the carbohydrates, and very quickly lost over 20 pounds. I became a true believer. I thrilled at eating eggs again, steak, and delectable desserts of sugar-free cheesecake with nut crust and chocolate truffles. "This is too good to be true," I exclaimed to myself—and to anyone else who would listen. "I am enjoying my favorite foods, can eat to satiation, and never have to feel hungry." I even found my cholesterol went down—and it hadn't been high in the first place.

I became convinced that Atkins was a modern hero who had single-handedly bucked the medical establishment. It had erroneously foisted low-fat diets upon us, only to yield the horrendous obesity problem we battle today. I persuaded a physician friend, and he began to tentatively recommend the Atkins diet to his patients. I enthusiastically initiated other friends with a sample of my Atkins-style, nut crust cheesecake!

But then something familiar happened: I reached a plateau and couldn't lose more than the initial 20 pounds. But at least I could maintain that loss and wasn't gaining. Then something worse happened: Almost imperceptibly, I began to follow the way of all flesh and the diet slipped away from me. Through bad times and good times, my eating increased and the pounds followed. Even though I biked long distances several times weekly, I regained all the weight I had lost. After a magnificent cruise in the Caribbean, with food that to my "hungry" eyes surpassed the islands' beauty, I added an additional 10 pounds during one week. I climbed ashore with an increased girth that topped out at 230 pounds, more than my weight before the diet. Sound familiar?

My bubble of enthusiasm burst and I had to face the fact that I had been wrong. I reverted to thinking that perhaps, as some believe, I was ruled by a biological set point that could only be fooled temporarily. My ability to apply a generally strong willpower to dieting had failed me yet again. The long-awaited epiphany from my client had turned out to be a false prophecy. He and his wife also regained the weight they had lost—and then some.

The truth is simply this: In the long run, diets alone don't work. Not the low fat diet, not the Grapefruit Diet, not the Atkins diet, not the "Next Diet," whatever it may be. The English scriptwriter Dennis Norden summed it up best: "There was only one occasion in my life when I put myself on a strict diet and I can tell you, hand over heart, it was the most miserable afternoon I have ever spent."

Is there any hope, I wondered, for the hopelessly overweight? There must be some solution. It simply didn't make sense that so many would be doomed to the myriad medical problems associated with obesity. This is not the way it was intended to be. This cannot be part of the cosmic plan. There must be an answer.

Eventually, I had a breakthrough—through a combination of confrontation and awareness. On a walk through the woods with a dear friend, the conversation turned to addiction. "Of all the problems I've had, addiction hasn't been one," I asserted.

My friend, who knew me well, gently suggested otherwise: "But you *use* food."

The notion that food was comforting to me was hardly new. My Jewish upbringing revolved around food: It meant celebration, family connection, and love. I recall the double-thick, extra-lean corned beef sandwiches that my father prepared lovingly and brought home Sunday nights from the New York deli where he worked to supplement his government job. The family gathered around the TV to watch Ed Sullivan—and ate.

But the notion that I was "using" food the way an addict uses a drug hit me with harsh clarity: I was addicted to food. I am an observant Jew, and I realized that if I was addicted to a substance, I was not dedicated to God with my entire self. Traditional Judaism teaches that you should "love the Lord your God with all your heart, with all your soul, and with all your power." If I let something other than God control me, my allegiance was divided. It occurred to me that we are taught to emulate our holy role models. I was certain that this was not the way our great prophet Moses would eat, nor his saintly sister, Miriam. The sages taught that we should be exceedingly humble because Moses was exceeding humble, and that we should emulate him.

I realized that there was something unholy about my use of food. With this awareness, I turned away from diets and towards God. I became intrigued about whether the Bible would provide clues to how Moses and Miriam ate so that we could follow their model. I re-discovered the long known, but rarely applied, solution to the intractable problem of being overweight—*Eating with holiness*. As I learned more, I discovered that this ancient wisdom is contained in the Bible and traditional spiritual practices rooted in Kabbalah. Although it is a simple truth, it has remained a "secret" for two reasons: First, for centuries the teachings of the Kabbalah were considered too esoteric for most people and were shared with only a small group of initiates. Second, for psychological reasons, people prefer not to talk about linking eating to holiness: They want to eat according to their own desires rather than follow God's will. Once this secret was revealed to me and became alive, I began losing weight easily—even joyfully—and with mounting confidence that something truly different was happening this time.

The problem is that during the obesity explosion of the last half-century, we have been desperately looking in the wrong direction for a solution. A notable exception is the 12-step program for weight loss. The originators of this program brilliantly intuited that a spiritual void and the need to turn to a Higher Power are at the core of disorders of desire, such as alcoholism and food addiction. But most modern strategies become preoccupied with diet—with *what* we eat. This preoccupation directs our gaze downward towards the earth where food grows rather than upward towards the source of the food itself—towards God and the deep connection between body and spirit, between eating and holiness.

The idea of Holy Eating was crystallizing. As I shed the first 25 pounds, many friends began to notice and comment, "You look great. How did you do it? I need to lose some weight too." This time I initially declined to start bubbling about my new enthusiasm. "I am not prepared to discuss it," I demurred. Being a psychotherapist, I would have loved to help. But I had learned that the more I spoke to convince others, the less likely it was that I was secure in my own practices. At this early stage, I felt this new approach was between God and me. Also, I didn't want to waste my friends' time with yet another intriguing—but short-lived—way to lose weight. After all, I could have paraphrased Mark Twain's comment on quitting smoking: "Losing weight is easy: I have done it dozens of times." Before I spoke out, I needed to see whether I would maintain the new weight.

The turning point came when I realized that I was focusing more on a closer relationship with God and less on food, or even on the gratifying weight loss itself. These became secondary benefits, not the preoccupations they used to be. When people who are dieting share a meal, they tend to talk *ad nauseam* about food: what they eat, what they don't eat, how this diet is really the one. They are still obsessed with food, as I was.

As more weight came off, the same good friends kept approaching me. When they asked a third time, I could no longer turn them away. "If you are really interested," I now replied, "let's sit down and talk for an hour or so. I am ready to share the secret." I was surprised that some people were able to grasp the idea of Holy Eating and make it work after as little as a single hour of discussion—and go on to lose 10, 15, even 25 pounds. But most needed a more intensive program.

While the core concept of Holy Eating continued guiding me toward both spiritual and physical transformation, I formed the idea of writing this book to share my experience with the many people seeking a solution. At this time, the spiritual leader of my community told me he had been cleaning his office and found a book that belonged to me. He had no idea why he had it and I did not recall giving it to him. But it had my name on it.

The book, *Jewish Spiritual Practices*, by Yitzchak Buxbaum is a treasure trove derived from Kabbalah and Chassidic (pietistic) sources that aims to elevate everyday activities by infusing them with spirituality. One chapter dealt with eating and inspired me to develop some of the strategies included here. Although Buxbaum does not apply these eating concepts to weight loss specifically, this volume indicates that there is nothing new in the approach that I describe here. Some of these ideas have been followed for hundreds of years, others no doubt for thousands. But today more than ever there is a need to apply them specifically to weight loss.

Happily, the wisdom of Kabbalah is, for the first time in history, becoming more widely available. For the past 200 years, the secrets of the Kabbalah have been distilled and revealed to the average person. Increasingly, non-Jews are also turning to this source of time-tested Jewish spiritual wisdom for guidance about how to live. I recall a popular New York advertisement for Levy's rye bread that showed smiling, multi-cultural individuals holding a large sandwich with a caption stating: "You don't have to be Jewish to enjoy Levy's Real Jewish Rye." Similarly, you don't have to be Jewish to benefit from Holy Eating because the universal teachings are totally consistent with the major world religions that grew out of Judaism.

But why look to Jews for insight into how to eat? The impression exists that many religious Jews are overweight. In fact, a Purdue University study found that obesity is associated with higher levels of religious participation for Jews and non-Jews alike. When the findings are broken down by creed, however, they show that Jews actually had a lower body-mass index than other religious groups. Nevertheless, this general finding seems to run counter to the concept of Holy Eating. Yet I believe that, paradoxically, it is totally consistent. As we shall see, food plays a dominant role in many biblical stories, from the first days of creation to the Exodus from Egypt. Food has been at the center of religious rituals from ancient sacrifices to contemporary celebrations. The problem is that for many religious, family-oriented individuals, food is an important celebratory focus, but the strong connection between the ritual and the spirituality has been severed.

This schism is dangerous. Religious practices and the cultural traditions that grow around them strongly orient the observant person toward food in order to sanctify it and elevate the experience of eating. But if the food loses its link to the spiritual realm, the eating behavior can descend to a place that is even lower than the norm. The higher something rises, the lower it can fall—if its spiritual momentum is not sustained.

The spirit of religious people gravitates to the important task of rectifying the split between soul and body that occurred in the Garden of Eden. According to biblical commentators, Adam was created originally outside the garden and God had to persuade him to enter and cultivate it. Adam was reluctant to give up his worldly attachments and enter this Paradise. The serpent enticed both Adam and Eve to engage in unholy eating by disobeying God's sole restrictive commandment to not eat from the Tree of Knowledge of Good and Evil. Through this act they acquired self-consciousness, were banished from the garden, and henceforth had to struggle with a separation between body and soul. Shame was born on that day and they covered their bodies. Adam and Eve's fateful choice left each of us struggling with continual temptations to follow the desires of our animal appetites rather than God's desire for us to be holy.

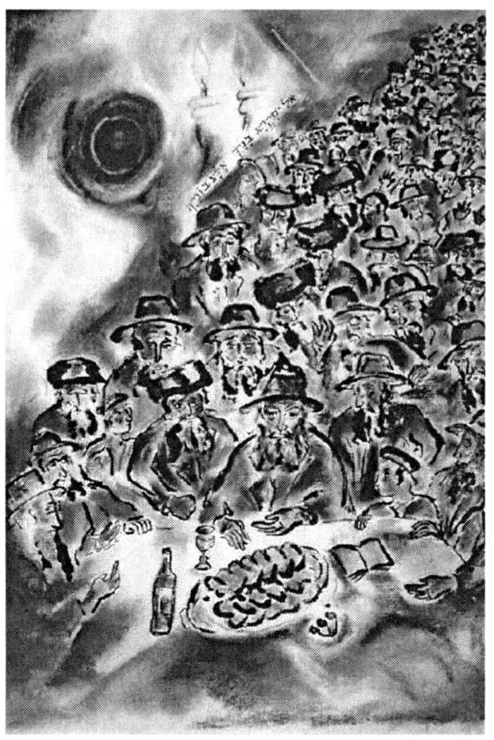

THE TABLE OF THE REBBE ("FARBRENGEN")

When a Chassidic Rebbe (Rabbi) conducts an official meal with his followers a lot of food is placed in front of him including a huge challah bread. He eats and is satisfied. What he leaves over (the majority of all this food, of course) is considered leftovers blessed by the rebbe. This is divided among his many followers who eat and are satisfied.

The human mission on Earth is to work towards re-entering the Garden by pursuing a path of holiness. Like Adam, a big part of us, our animal nature, remains reluctant. The journey begins, but does not end, with cultivating Holy Eating. This is why the first story in biblical history involves eating and why food figures so prominently in Judaism and many world religions. There is a quip that summarizes the history of the Jewish people: "They tried to kill us, we won, let's eat." The problem for our society, for both religious and non-religious people alike, is that the final phrase should read, "Let's eat *with holiness." The soul of eating has been removed from the act of eating, leaving only bodily appetites—and the resulting obesity epidemic.*

Spirituality inspires people to seek unity and heal whatever is broken—in this case, how we eat. So religious people in particular have an above-average interest in food and celebratory feasts, which can cause the paradoxical problem of overeating when the higher purpose is obscured. People who sit down to weekly Sabbath meals or frequent religious feasts face more regular temptation than those who don't. If they lose their focus on faith at meals, they can grow obese. But if they unify the spiritual with the physical, they can make their meals holy, elevating the food, themselves and the world.

I have published many scientific papers on positive thinking and cognitive-behavioral therapy strategies for treating depression, anxiety and stress. I learned from my scientific research that motivation is driven by both positive and negative experiences, by the carrot and the stick. Pursuing holiness should be primarily a positive and joyful journey, filled with song and dance, celebrating God's love. That's the carrot. But I have recently seen too many of my friends and revered teachers perish from health problems that may have been brought on or worsened by excess weight. That's the stick.

Although my mother had reduced her weight after she developed health problems, I now believe that her 10-year descent into Alzheimer's disease was triggered by a period of active diabetes and related mini-strokes. With her death fresh in my heart, I wrote this book with the hope that it might help others to avoid unnecessary suffering from illness and premature loss of life—that it might instead lead them to an enhancement of physical well-being, self-esteem and spiritual growth.

This book will help you understand and internalize the concept of Holy Eating so that it comes alive with spiritual force. The book will guide you through practical steps toward experiencing the ultimate pleasures of Holy Eating, with its benefits of reduced shame and improved fitness, beauty, and health. Unlike the majority of weight loss books, *Holy Eating* will not—and need not—tell you specifically what to eat. No particular food groups need to be avoided completely, but all must be eaten with holiness. This often means eating certain foods in smaller quantities, but instead of deprivation you will feel abundance and satisfaction. If you have a food plan you like, you can continue with it. Holy Eating may be the only missing ingredient that your diet needs to make it work.

By altering the way you eat, you will not merely derive health benefits or weight loss. You will grow spiritually and transform yourself into a better person. In fact, Holy Eating turns the entire process of dieting upside down. You are first and foremost embarking on a spiritual journey that happens to result in what I call *weight transformation* rather than weight loss. As you will see, your weight is not merely "lost" since the energy stored in fat cells is transformed into increased activity, positive self-esteem, greater health, and longevity, all of which enable you to do more good in the world. Increasing light through good deeds is the ultimate purpose of a spiritual life. Eating is the starting point and the repeatedly traveled road on this journey. Please join me and you will surely reach your destination. Let there be more light in your spirit and more lightness in your body.

PART I:
Transform Yourself Through Holy Eating

Chapter 1

◆ ◆ ◆ ◆ ◆ ◆ ◆ ◆ ◆ ◆ ◆ ◆ ◆ ◆

God Wants You Holy, Healthy—and Trim

"You shall be holy, because I, the Lord your God, am holy..."
—Leviticus 19:2

"I have placed life and death before you, blessing and curse; and you shall choose life, so that you will live..."
—Deuteronomy 30:19

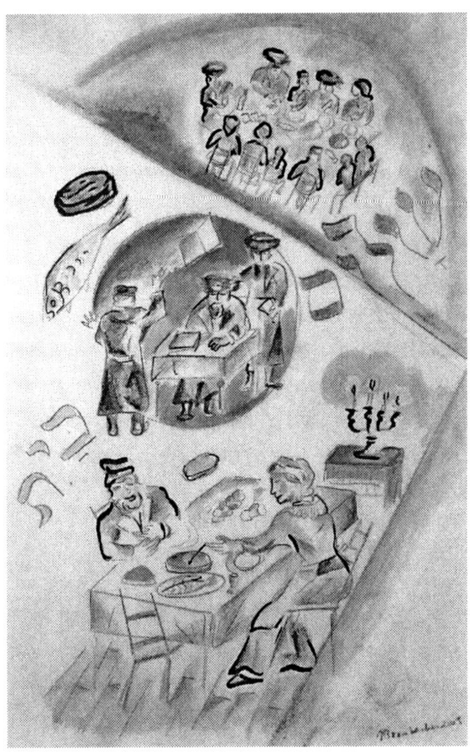

Peace in the Home (Shalom Bayis)

I recall joking many years ago to a friend at a health club, "If I had only lost one pound per year for the past 25 years, I would be at my ideal weight." A more than modest goal, but one I never achieved. Instead, the dial on the scale gradually shifted in the opposite direction, until it peaked at 50 pounds overweight. Anyone should be able to lose a pound a year, or even a pound a month. But therein lies the rub. Despite great desire and billions spent on diets and supplements, most people gain rather than lose.

Two-thirds of American adults are either overweight or obese. Of these 130 million people struggling with weight problems, most have tried dieting. But according to studies published in respected journals, most dieters fail to lose much weight, and the vast majority of those who do gain it back within 5 years. This trend will only worsen as a consequence of the plague of childhood obesity now gripping the nation. The continual proliferation of new diets only proves their inadequacy. Some overweight people have turned to drastic surgical procedures. Now that FDA-approved appetite suppressants have become available, more people will abandon the traditional value of temperance.

Why is it so easy to gain weight and so hard to shed pounds? What makes failed self-regulation of body weight a national epidemic? Is there any force powerful enough to counter overwhelming cravings for food and the weight gain that follows?

You are probably reading this book because you personally haven't discovered this powerful force and are still overweight. You are searching for an answer. You may unfortunately be experiencing or worrying about developing weight-related health problems, such as high cholesterol, hypertension, heart disease, diabetes, joint problems, chronic back pain, or some forms of cancer. A recent study published in the Proceedings of the National Academy of Sciences indicates that insulin resistance in brain cells can affect how they function, causing some of the biochemical changes typical of Alzheimer's disease. This finding suggests that Alzheimer's may be considered a form of Type 3 diabetes, creating yet new worries about being overweight.

There is an Answer

Thank God, there is an answer: **Holy Eating**. To put it simply: God made all parts of creation with intelligence and love, with harmony and good form. God intended all of us to become our best and true selves and to achieve our mission in life. This intended ideal includes both character refinement as well as a certain bodily form. If you are overweight or obese, this intended form is NOT what you see today when you look in the mirror. God designed each individual to be within an optimal weight range; if you carry excess weight that is not the result of illness, this optimal number is not what you see when you get on the scale.

God wants you to be holy, healthy—and trim. As we will see, the Bible makes it crystal clear that God desires us to be holy, to take care of our health, and yes, to also control our food intake and avoid excess body weight. Before examining these sources, consider the truth of these assertions and the logic of the conclusion:

1. God loves you.
2. God wants you to be healthy.
3. Obesity is associated with illness, not health.
4. *Therefore, God wants you to be trim.*

God loves every part of creation and at a fundamental level accepts you unconditionally as you are. Yet, scientific research continues to demonstrate beyond doubt that being overweight or obese can seriously damage health. So, it follows logically that *God also wants you to find your optimal weight.*

Most people readily agree that God wants us to be both holy and healthy, but does God actually focus on our weight? For an answer, let's look at the story of Moses. As the end of Moses' life drew near, God appeared to him in a pillar of cloud and told him to write a song and teach it to the children of Israel, to "place it in their mouth." (Note the figure of speech!) The very first point that God instructs Moses to include concerns food and overeating:

> "When I will bring it [the people of Israel] to the land that I have sworn to its ancestors—that flows with milk and honey—it will eat and be satisfied, and *it will become obese* [italics added]; it will turn to other gods and serve them, it will provoke Me, and break My covenant."[1]

The Bible states clearly here that obesity represents a serious turning away from God and a potential breach of the spiritual bond with the divine. God chose eating as our initial struggle because it is the primary battleground for self-control that is required for a spiritual life.

We need to clarify what this means. Optimal body weight means a body that is well proportioned, with the appropriate amount of fat that suits each body type. It does not mean overly thin or skinny. Preoccupation with excessive thinness is also inconsistent with Holy Eating because it is not conducive to health and indicates an improper relationship with both God and food. The word "trim" connotes removing excess, as well as being fit, healthy, and in good physical shape. Moderation is possible. *In this sense, God wants you to be trim.*

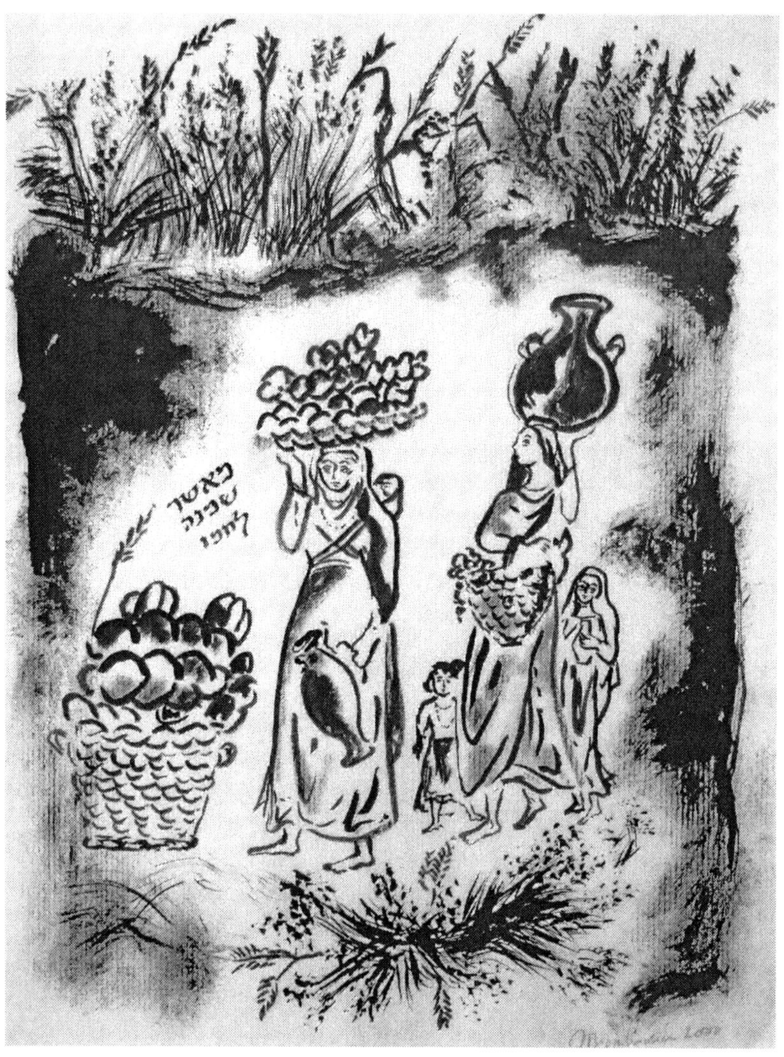

The Tribe of Asher

The tribe of Asher was blessed in the Bible with abundant food: "Out of Asher his bread shall have richness, and he shall yield royal delicacies." (Genesis: 49:20).

Once you fully understand and adopt Holy Eating, you can achieve this goal. You will also have taken a major step towards lifelong health—both physical and spiritual. The quest for Holy Eating requires a commitment to grow and to reflect about God, food, and yourself in different ways. But once you grasp the deep connections among these elements, eating properly will soon become easier than you ever imagined.

No advanced knowledge of Jewish texts is required to employ this approach. The only requirement is that you begin with a spiritual awareness, however faint, of a force or higher power in the universe that transcends your self and operates with greater strength than natural forces alone. If you have a strong belief in God and already turn to God for connection, inspiration, and support, your journey will be smoother because you will grasp the concepts more readily. But if you have read this far, your interest in spirituality is strong enough to grow to the level needed for success. As you will see later, the earliest stage of the human quest for spirituality can be found in one's relationship to God and food. *The physical, mundane act of eating is actually an ideal place to start or renew your spiritual journey.*

Later I will provide strategies drawn from both spiritual and psychological sources to sharpen your focus and elevate your eating. But the first step is to develop a more intimate knowledge of the concept of Holy Eating itself.

Holy Eating

According to Holy Eating, the answer lies in returning eating behavior to its proper context: For humans, eating is a spiritual act. Eating with spirituality involves a recognition that one is partaking of the divine gift of food that comes from God for the purpose of maintaining a healthy body to fulfill one's life task. For animals, eating is regulated by instinct alone, and animals in their natural habitat will rarely eat to excess. They do not have free choice in this domain any more than in other aspects of existence.

But when humans lose connection with the spiritual nature of eating, they fall out of harmony with God's will and the natural order of things. When life was simpler, this connection came more naturally. With the advent of technology, affluence and fast food this bond became more remote and tenuous. Rabbi Dr. Abraham Twerski, renowned authority on addictive disorders, has often said that addictions can best be understood as a futile attempt to fulfill a spiritual void with some physical substance. Soul hunger can be confused with physical appetite. We are witnessing an epidemic of what Dr. Twerski calls "SDS," Spiritual Deficiency Syndrome. Spiritual voids can be filled only with spirit, so no amount of food is sufficient to satisfy and consumption becomes excessive.

Once you adopt Holy Eating, you will shift your focus from physical metabolism to what I call "*spiritual metabolism*,"—a process that frees you from the preoccupation with food and diets and replaces it with a deeply satisfying connection with God. You will realize that your excess hunger for food stems from your hidden hunger for spirituality and God. Spiritual metabolism is both a metaphor and a reality. Physical metabolism involves chemical reactions that provide the energy and nutrients to sustain the life of the body. In the realm of what psychologist William James called the "reality of the unseen," spiritual metabolism creates the nutrients needed to animate and elevate the soul, which in turn interacts with and satisfies the body. As with the mind-body connection, there is a spirit-body connection.

Everyone is familiar with the maxim "you are what you eat," and that's true, to a great extent. Many religions prescribe and prohibit certain foods, and nutritionists have demonstrated that foods differ in their health value. But once you are eating the right foods, your humanity is defined less by what you eat than by *how* you eat. Different peoples thrive on various diets ranging from vegetarian to carnivorous. For Westerners, bread is a staple, whereas the Chinese depend on rice. Although a certain balance of nutrients is required, the digestive process is a great equalizer that can take a variety of culinary inputs and transform them into adequate nutrition. But every great culture has developed elaborate customs that govern both what is eaten and how a meal is prepared and consumed.

Holy Eating focuses on the spiritual meaning and the manner in which you eat. It is not another diet that emphasizes a biological theory about how certain foods will break your food addiction and keep weight off. Holy Eating begins with God as the prime motivator, not with diets or calories—or even your inner self and willpower. Holy Eating takes you beyond *self*-management to *God*-management. The focus of Holy Eating involves understanding what God wants from you in life, and, most importantly, the way in which God wants you to eat. The path to eternal weight loss is to discover *how* God wanted Moses and Miriam to eat, and to internalize this attitude and manner of eating.

Religious and spiritually oriented people unfamiliar with Kabbalah will find these traditional teachings new to them, but will quickly be able to appreciate the profound truth they contain. People following a 12-step program do not draw directly on any specific religion but will find this approach consistent with their spiritual principles. Holy Eating is especially helpful at Step 11: "[We] Sought to improve our conscious contact with God *as we understood Him*, praying only for knowledge of His will for us and the power to carry that out." But for most people, this book will reveal an open secret that is typically concealed: God cares deeply about how you eat.

Towards a Spiritual-Psychological Integration

Holy Eating integrates powerful spiritual beliefs with modern cognitive-behavioral methods of change. For decades, psychologists have developed weight management programs based on scientific studies for people who should be motivated to lose weight, such as diabetics and coronary patients. Despite millions of dollars of research on participants coping with life-threatening conditions, these programs have been only marginally successful because people often regain whatever weight was lost. Neither psychology nor medicine alone, despite outstanding success in overcoming many disorders, has been able to successfully manage excess eating.

In our era, many overweight people are themselves religious. Today, religious people may benefit from more structure and tools to successfully apply their spiritual concepts to healthful eating. At the same time, psychological approaches without spirituality lack sufficiently powerful content to consistently control eating. Holy Eating offers an integrated approach that brings together eternal spiritual principles with modern cognitive-behavioral strategies. Although the ancient spiritual practices that have successfully guided our ancestors for millennia contain implicit tools that are "cognitive-behavioral" in nature, many spiritually oriented people today will find it useful to have these techniques dressed in more contemporary clothing.

Judith Beck, Director of the Beck Institute of Cognitive Therapy, developed a standard, secular program based on 20 years of helping people lose weight by changing how they think. The program teaches the dieter that instead of thinking, "I enjoy spontaneous munching. I don't want to stop eating standing up," they should think, "I need to sit down to eat. When I eat standing up, I just don't notice what I'm eating." Although promising, cognitive-behavioral approaches alone that focus on rational, non-spiritual thoughts have not demonstrated sufficient change power to control excess eating. Most dieters have probably experienced expressing rational thoughts such as, "I shouldn't eat a second helping", even while shoveling the next spoonful into their mouths. Holy Eating offers an option that harnesses the power of cognitive-behavioral psychology, but avoids the limitations of relying exclusively on these techniques.

Rabbi Dr. Abraham Twerski, noted above, has said that Judaism is a very cognitive-behavioral religion. This is because it places heavy emphasis on correct thinking, stresses the importance of proper action, and offers daily practices or tools to achieve these goals. But unlike psychological approaches such as cognitive therapy that rely on the power of the rational mind alone, Judaism and religions derived from it offer a divine source for the cognitions and behaviors that are practiced.

Holy Eating offers what I refer to as "high octane cognitions," thoughts that pack a powerful punch because of their specific derivation from God. For example, instead of a person merely thinking, "I need to sit down while eating," which may not control behavior, Holy Eating offers a deeper context for this thought that draws on a spiritual value system. The Talmud instructs that we shouldn't eat meals while standing because this is how animals eat and that a person who eats in the street would not be worthy to serve as a reliable witness in court. The same thought—"I need to sit down"—when derived from a higher authority, provides the spiritual "octane" that empowers a person to actually listen and sit down. She is listening not only to herself, but also to the voice of God. Thoughts control behavior more effectively if one firmly believes they come from a higher source.

The Quest for Spiritual Transformation

The Talmud, the commentary on the Bible, advises us that because all comes from God, we must thank God with joy for the bad things that happen to us as well as for the good. Surely if this is possible, we can at least learn to eat less food with joyfulness, without a sense of constant deprivation and strain. Holy Eating is the path to this transcendent experience. With Holy Eating, you never have to feel hungry again. You will learn to experience a healthy and hearty appetite, but not confuse it with hunger. You will learn to replace deprivation with gratitude and satisfaction.

There's a story about an honest man who sought answers as to why he was suffering. He was advised to visit Rabbi Zusya, a poor man himself who lived in a hillside hovel with his family and knew many hardships. When the man told the Rabbi he had come to learn why people suffer, Rabbi Zusya replied with bewilderment, "I don't know why they sent you to me. I have never known a day of suffering in my life." Similarly, I can say that since adopting Holy Eating, I have never experienced a moment of hunger while losing considerable weight. Reducing physical desires so they are experienced in a balanced, moderate way draws you closer to God. Elevating these desires into love of God and directing this love to others in the form of caring, compassion, giving, and generosity transforms you into a better person.

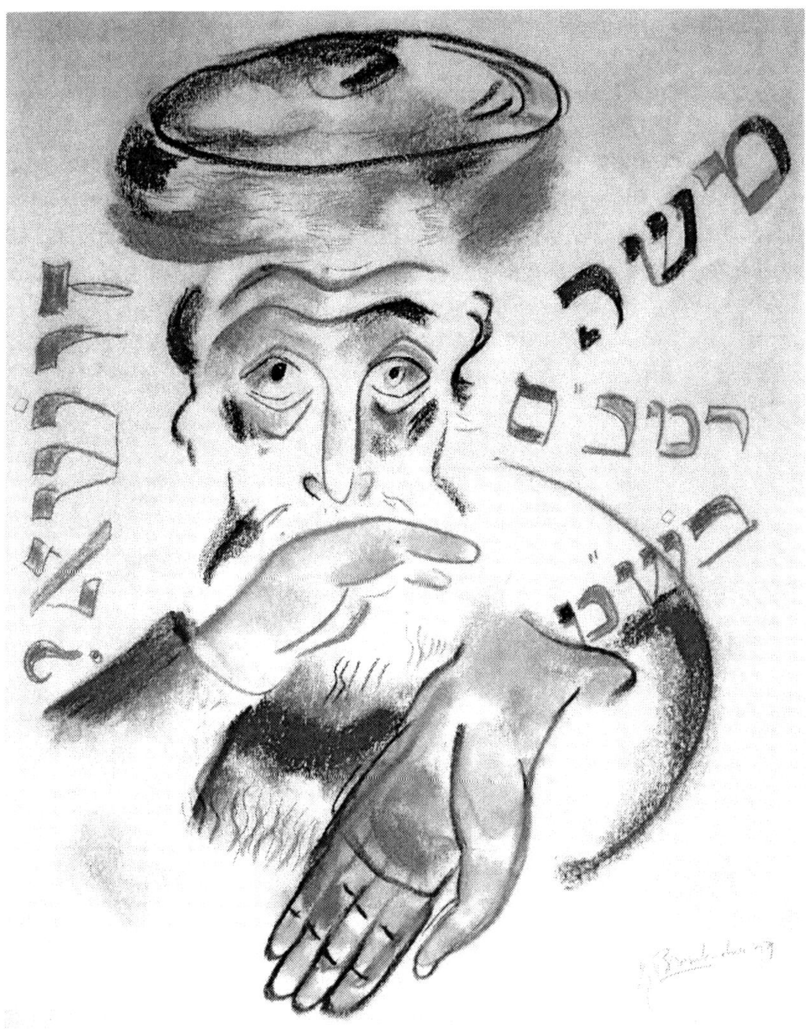

Rabbi Zusya

Rabbi Zusya considered what the Heavenly Court might ask him after he died. "They will not ask me if I lived like Moshe Rabbenu (Moses), or like Rambam (Maimonides), or like the Baal Shem Tov. No, they will ask me: 'Did you live like Zusya?"

Losing weight is a secondary gain that results from this transformational process. In Holy Eating you will not focus primarily on weight, looking better, or even being healthier. Focusing too heavily on looking better promotes vanity, which will not sustain your motivation over the long run. If you focus exclusively on health or longevity, the outcomes are too distant. The primary focus of Holy Eating is the knowledge of God's will for you *at this moment and at every moment.* While working with people on Holy Eating, I am amazed how infrequently we discuss weight loss or food—and yet the weight comes off. Does this sound too good to be true? Rather, it is too true not to be good. It is a simple and beautiful truth for those who take the step of connecting faith to the routine of daily eating.

Freedom from Food Slavery Through Serving the Right Master

Is Holy Eating merely another healthy "lifestyle choice" or is it what God commands us to do? I believe it has the force of a commandment. The biblical exhortation that "You shall be holy, because I, the Lord your God, am holy" is all-encompassing, covering everything from how to awaken in the morning to how to tie one's shoes. If so, vital life issues such as health and eating must also come under the purview of God's will for us to conduct ourselves with holiness.

This view is supported by biblical and Talmudic sources culled by Rabbi Reuven Bulka in a useful volume entitled *Judaism and Pleasure.* When God created Man from the dust of the ground, "He blew into his nostrils the soul of life and he became a living being." [2]

The commentary explains the verse's meaning: "The soul that I [God] have placed in you, sustain it."[3] The blessing of life brings with it the responsibility to care for both the body and soul. The Bible further instructs us to "Be exceedingly heedful of your selves."[4] This passage refers to the obligation of self-preservation. Most biblical commandments simply instruct us about what to do without further qualification. Here we are told to be "*exceedingly*" heedful, emphasizing the importance of being vigilant and unwavering in our pursuit of health.

The Bible tells us directly that God wants us to be well. A commentary explains that the verse, "And God will remove from you all sickness,"[5] indicates that our personal choices play a role in fulfilling or defying God's will: "It is from you [within your control] that sickness should not befall you."[6] Although it says God will remove sicknesses and that we play a role in controlling our health, the relationship between faith and health is complex. There are some trim people who succumb to illness and some overweight ones who do not. We cannot always understand completely why these things happen.

Nevertheless, we will see that many additional spiritual sources make it obligatory to cultivate physical health and refrain from harmful activity. We now have scientific knowledge that overeating is bad for health, as we have seen, we are instructed to be "exceedingly heedful" in pursuing self-preservation. It therefore follows logically that avoiding excess weight must be viewed not merely as a lifestyle choice, but as a holy commandment.

Since most want to be totally free, this can be a challenge to accept. I recall a formative experience that occurred on a cool autumn day during my first year of living according to Jewish law, which can be demanding. Observant Jews are not allowed to use hot tap water on the Sabbath, because creative work is forbidden and the water heater might ignite a "fire" to replenish the hot water in its tank. As my ancestors did before me in the desert (although they kvetched mostly about food issues), I was muttering to God in front of the bathroom mirror about this indignity: "Why do we have to be so uncomfortable? If I just use a small amount of warm water, it won't empty the tank. We are supposed to live by Your laws, not suffer from them."

Suddenly a loud explosion halted my litany of complaints. The room went dark.

"Okay, okay, God. I accept Your law. I'll use cold water and I won't complain!"

Apparently the light bulb above the bathroom mirror had burst at just the right moment. I can't say whether God had timed this event for my personal benefit, but religious people believe that everything happens for a reason. I hope that, in the case of your eating, some light bulb will flash on for you. When you link eating properly to God's will, everything becomes much simpler.

Letting God take command makes change easier because God's will is so much stronger than our own, particularly in the battle against overeating. Sadly, many people have negative images of an authoritarian or punishing God, which makes them resist surrendering. But eating in general and Holy Eating in particular is a blessing originating from God's loving kindness and nurturance. If you can receive this imperative as lovingly given, it gains extraordinary force. Submission to God's will is both liberating and elevating. A paradoxical tenet of faith is that serving God, as the only Master, frees one from enslavement to other tyrants—including food.

Choose Life

Something deep within you yearns to be healthy and fit, perhaps for the first time in decades. On an intuitive level you know that being trim is better for you. Since God gave you free choice it's ultimately up to you to choose. Although weight gain feels as though it's out of your control, the truth is that for most people overeating is a choice: It depends on how you eat. So you can instead choose to become healthy and trim. *You can choose life.*

Goal-Setting. Decisions can be weak and fleeting or strong and enduring. Cognitive-behavioral psychology recommends becoming specific about your goal in order to clarify and strengthen your choice. Precisely what does it mean for your body to be healthy and trim? One answer, and the most commonly used, comes from the National Institute of Health's body mass index (BMI) guidelines. The simplest way to compute your BMI is to use a BMI calculator online at the National Institute of Health website at www.nhlbisupport.com/bmi. Or you can calculate your BMI with this formula: weight (lb.) / $[\text{height (in)}]^2$ x 703, which means divide your weight in pounds by your height in inches squared, and multiply by the number 703. Normal weight as defined by the National Institute of Health is a BMI between 18.5-24.9, overweight is 25-29.9, and obese is 30 or greater.

In using the BMI index, consider your body type. God loves diversity and created several body types: Some are large-boned and muscular, some round with soft body tissue, and others slightly built, angular and naturally thin. All these people may have trim bodies if they lack excess body fat, but each will look different and have optimal weights that fall at different places within the BMI range.

Another way to clarify your target goal is to measure your body fat directly, using readily available body composition scales that show what percentage of your body is fat, muscle mass, or water (see www.tanita.com for a low-cost option). Depending on age and sex, healthy body fat percentage can vary from as little as 8% of total body weight in a young man in his 20's to 36% in a woman in her 70's. Generally, women have about 10% more body fat than men do, and the amount gradually increases between 3-5% from early to late adulthood for both sexes.

Remember that two-thirds of Americans are out of the normal range, whether measured by BMI calculation or body fat level. Because so many people are overweight, our vision of a desirable weight is skewed. Often people tend to overestimate their optimal weight, especially men.

If you want a quick estimate of your optimal body weight, think back to a time after age 18 when you were at your ideal weight. (If you were overweight from childhood, you will need to rely on the BMI calculator.)

Take that weight and add 5% to it, and you will get a target figure to aim for. For example, in college I weighed between 165 and 175 pounds. If I add 5% to the higher figure, I get 175 x .05 = 9 lbs. Since 175 + 9 = 184, I would target between 175 and 184 pounds; I'd be content simply remaining at the upper limit of 184.

Motivation. Once you have established a target weight, write it down and set it aside for now. As in sports, you can't look ahead to playing the championship; you need to focus on winning one game at a time. You want to concentrate on clarifying why you want to lose weight and transforming how you eat. The first step is to affirm that you do have a choice. But simply choosing is not enough—you must make a *strong* choice that has the force of conviction. To make a choice that packs power, first open your mind to imagine the positive—and negative—possibilities of the paths of continued weight gain versus weight loss. Now focus on the positive advantages of achieving your long-sought goal.

Ask yourself the ultimate motivational question: *Why* exactly do you want to lose weight? Think about this for a few moments and list the reasons below. Leave the first line blank. We will come back to it in a moment.

____

____

____

____

____

____

____

____

Most people say they want to lose weight because of health:

"I want to be healthy."
"My blood pressure is elevated."
"I had a heart attack."
"Diabetes has set in."
"My physician told me I better lose weight or I'll need medication."

Some say they want to live longer for their children. Others want to feel better or more energetic, to feel less pain or fatigue. Many cite a wish to look more attractive.

Were your reasons similar? They are all sensible motivations to lose weight. But each of these motives is incomplete. The problem is that while people say they want to lose weight because of high blood pressure or aching knees, when they begin a meal they are no longer thinking about their heart or legs—they are thinking about their stomachs. Most of the time, serious health conditions have only distant consequences, so even sincere and motivated dieters give in to the more immediate urge to satisfy their appetite.

The problem is that these reasons for weight loss depend on only personal willpower and the latest diet. *They lack the essential active ingredient that transcends the personal self: God.*

I have asked many people why they want to lose weight. Interestingly, I have yet to encounter a single person, even among the most religious, who mentioned the most powerful source of motivation and change. No one has spontaneously answered that he or she wanted to lose weight out of a belief that *this is what God wants.* This is not merely a peripheral truth, but a central reality of human existence and a fundamental aspect of spiritual life.

The essence of Holy Eating—and the secret to eternal weight loss— is a shift from self-focused to God-focused motivation. When you become convinced of this, go back to the blank first line of your reasons to lose weight and add: "Because God wants me to be trim." Congratulations if you already included this.

Clearly, there is no quick fix for weight loss and no shortcut to spirituality. Holy Eating challenges you to engage in activities necessary for spiritual growth: learning, thinking, and undertaking or strengthening daily spiritual practices. A central tenet of both Judaism and cognitive psychology is that thinking has the power to control how we behave and feel. Spiritual transformation requires a profound shift in thinking about food–what cognitive therapy calls *cognitive restructuring.* For this reason it is important that you spend time contemplating the biblical and kabbalistic sources in the following sections that form the basis of Holy Eating. Ideas have power to transform the world—especially ideas from God. Taste and digest these delicacies and your hunger will be transformed.

I guarantee that if you understand and apply these spiritual principles daily at each meal, you will find this a true and certain path that will elevate your soul while diminishing your waistline.

CHAPTER 2

◆ ◆ ◆ ◆ ◆ ◆ ◆ ◆ ◆ ◆ ◆ ◆ ◆ ◆

The Tree of Knowledge and God-Conscious Eating

"Then the eyes of both of them were opened
and they realized that they were naked."
—Genesis 3:7

"It was a fig—the thing that had caused their ruin
was also their rectification."
—Talmud, Sanhedrin 76a

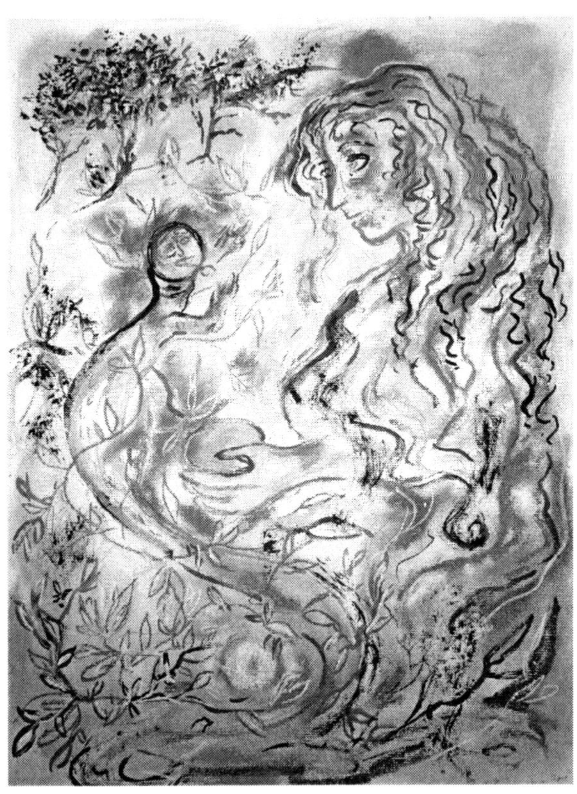

EVE AND THE SNAKE

Put away the diet books. Step back from the obsession with weight loss, calories, and carbohydrates—the preoccupation with food itself. Take a look at the big picture—the historical view, reaching back to the beginning of human history, as recounted in the Bible. It's the dawn of the sixth day since the Creation. God has completed the physical universe, including all the plants and animals. He sculpts Adam out of earth and Eve from his side. Just hours later, the first dramatic event of human history occurs, with consequences that reverberate to this day. What is this momentous event?

A hint: It has to do with food.

According to *midrash*, or scholarly elaborations of biblical stories, as the blessed couple awakens to a splendid dawn on their first morning, they are ready to celebrate the first Sabbath. They are enveloped in purity and holiness, at one with God and themselves. Their body and soul are united in harmony. They have free range of the Garden of Eden—with a single restriction: They are forbidden to eat fruit from the tree of knowledge of good and evil. But Eve has noble aspirations. She wants to acquire knowledge so she can rise closer to God. The serpent shrewdly manipulates her, through both her sensual desires and her intellectual strivings. Eve tastes the forbidden fruit, but that's not enough. She wants her husband to share in her accomplishment. Adam trusts her and willingly eats.

Although positive desires motivate Adam and Eve, they have defied God. Their new knowledge alters their awareness of their bodies. They feel shame and cover themselves with fig leaves. The original unity of body and soul is severed. God banishes Adam and Eve from the Garden; they forfeit eternal life. From then on, Man must toil for his bread and Woman bear children in pain. All will eventually know death.

Soon after men and women were created, they committed the first sin: Unholy eating. God's first spiritual challenge to humankind does not involve prohibitions on murder, greed, dishonesty, or sloth, but rather rules regarding eating. Of course murder will follow as a close second when Cain kills Abel. Before long the people of Sodom and Gomorrah will decline into debauchery, culminating in the cleansing Flood. Disobedience and debauchery will continue to fill the dramatic pages of the Bible, but it all begins with eating.

Clearly God was particularly invested in the regulation of eating. Let's explore why. According to Rabbi David Aaron, the Bible teaches that God created the world so we could experience goodness, and the greatest goodness conceivable is connecting with God. We can bond with God by serving His purpose in creation, by doing what He wants us to do. Just as we feel connected when we do something for a friend, so we connect to God by serving Him. The term "holy" means exactly this: connection with God or devotion to serving God.

When we enjoy the fruits of this world for God's sake, for the sake of Heaven, we draw closer to God. We recognize that those fruits come as a gift, and we graciously accept them in the way God wants us to. According to Kabbalah, the joy of connecting to God yields the most profound and lasting pleasure in life—*holy pleasure.* The prototype of holy pleasure was the blissful unity enjoyed in the Garden of Eden by following God's commandment to taste all the luscious fruits of the world, except one. Eating when disconnected from God can titillate and satisfy our lust in the short term, but negative consequences follow; eating with *God-consciousness* yields a more transcendent and stable joy, minus the side effects.

When Adam and Eve ate from the tree of knowledge, they became confused in their orientation to pleasure. Instead of focusing on holy pleasure from eating to serve God, they craved the freedom of eating rebelliously. The Hebrew word for serpent is *nachash*, which means a blind, impulsive urge, like an instinctual drive. Before the first humans ate from the tree of knowledge, the unity between body and soul yielded a natural control of such urges, so that desires were balanced and holy.

Eating the forbidden fruit initiated not only self-consciousness but also the potential to be dominated by physical desires, especially by the appetite for food. Since God does not give us something we can't master, He also gave us self-awareness so we could make choices and exercise self-control. *The problem today is that we have the serpent's legacy of blind urges that are no longer naturally balanced, but we fail to use consciousness—the power of mind and soul—to master them.*

The outcome of Adam and Eve's disobedience was a fateful downshift from *God*-consciousness to *self*-consciousness, from an all-encompassing awareness of God to a narrow focus on the self. When we eat with God-consciousness, we experience a holy, ultimate pleasure from the joy of serving God and feeling connected to Him. But when we eat with only self-consciousness, we feel merely sensual pleasure that disconnects us from God and severs the bond between the physical and the spiritual. Such pleasure can indeed be intense, but it leads to over-indulgence, is fleeting, and culminates in shame.

Sarah Schneider observed that the great Kabbalist, Rabbi Tsadok HaKohen, made the fascinating point that Adam and Eve's sin was not so much *what* they ate but *how.*[7] The tree of knowledge of good and evil, Rabbi Tsadok says, was not a primarily a tree or a food, or even a thing at all. Rather, it was a *way* of eating that revealed how Adam and Eve engaged with the world.[8]

When a person grabs self-conscious pleasure from the world, s/he falls, at that moment, from God's consciousness. In Rabbi Tsadok's broader view, all personality imbalances and existential dissatisfactions have their root in this first sin of unholy eating. Everyone has an "eating disorder," for eating is more than simply taking food into one's mouth. All desires conceived not in the service of God—whether for possessions, sensual pleasures, honors, power, praise, or drugs—are forms of unholy eating or consuming that eventually lead to emotional pain or physical illness. That is why in the Bible unholy eating precedes all other acts of separating from God.

Rabbi Aaron, cited earlier, distinguishes between *having* pleasure and *receiving* pleasure. *Having* pleasure is pleasure for its own sake. It is devoid of a connection to anything transcendent and unconcerned about origins. The very expressions we use, such as "he had his pleasure…" or "she took pleasure in…," connote grasping. On the other hand, *receiving* pleasure emphasizes that the pleasure is rooted in the soul's desire to serve God, to experience transcendent joy that comes as a gift of God. One does not "have" or "take" but rather "receives" holy pleasure from the awareness that God is the ultimate source of all goodness, including sensual pleasure. That may be one reason that these spiritual secrets are called Kabbalah, which means "to receive or accept" – as in accepting traditional wisdom.

Because Adam and Eve had eaten the forbidden fruit, God told them, "The Earth has become cursed." This enduring curse fluctuates depending on how we relate to the physical world. Originally the physical and the spiritual were united, so all permitted pleasures were automatically enjoyed in holiness. Now the physical Earth and its derivatives are a curse when we let them remain separate from God. But we can transform the material world back into a blessing by engaging with it as a bridge to the spiritual—if we receive God's precious gifts with God-consciousness, rather than grabbing them out of self-consciousness. Purely physical eating fails to satisfy, leading to the need for more and more stimulation with the consequent gain in weight.

If we think about God when eating by saying blessings or grace over a meal, we transform the curse of materiality into a blessing. Each meal, indeed each bite and swallow, becomes another step toward rectifying the original sin of Adam and Eve by infusing spirituality into physicality and restoring their severed unity. In contrast, each act of unholy eating reinforces, ever so slightly, the original error in the Garden and widens the rift.

Unholy eating is where our troubles began. But each holy meal brings us a step closer to the garden of earthly bliss. This is why eating is so important to religious people and why it needs to be correctly understood and practiced.

A Well-Ordered Universe, A Well-Formed Body

"I provide knowledge of designs."
—Proverbs 8:12

Kabbalah teaches that the ultimate purpose of human life is to connect with—to receive—the divine. But this is not to disparage the mundane. Abraham Lincoln observed that common people are the best, since God created so many of them. Likewise, God must have loved the physical world, because he certainly made a lot of it. Look up at the sun-drenched sky on a clear day or the star-filled radiance of night. Contemplate for several moments the expansive universe and the idea of creation. Consider that God created the universe with divine intelligence, from the brightly colorful plants and birds to the inspiring complexity of the human brain.

The universe is called a *cosmos* because it is a well-balanced and harmonious whole. The sun rises in the East at predictable times throughout the seasons and sets regularly in the West. The planets follow geometric patterns as they orbit through the heavens and the stars are arranged in heavenly constellations. Many spiritual traditions have observed that Man is a microcosm of the macrocosm, a small version of a well-ordered universe.

Since everything comes from God, the entire created world is an expression of God's Mind. The task of humankind is to see this universal order and to align ourselves with it by bringing our mind and body into harmony with God's Divine Mind. When we are unified with God's will, the microcosm lines up with the macrocosm. Since the cosmos is constructed according to balance, this alignment establishes the proper balance in body and mind.

God has been called a geometrician because He gave mathematical form and proportion to every aspect of creation. Atoms maintain a specific number of electrons and protons. With a slight alteration atoms can change from inert to explosive, from benign to deadly. If the amount of oxygen in the atmosphere decreased even slightly, combustion would cease; if increased, the world would burn.

The body, too, must maintain delicate balances. For example, we breathe in oxygen and exhale carbon dioxide. This oxygen-carbon dioxide balance determines the pH levels in the blood. Overall pH levels can range from 0 to 14. But the blood pH level in a normal human must remain in an extremely narrow range, between 7.35 - 7.45, with the ideal level being exactly 7.4. Below or above this balance point yields symptoms and disease. Even a small change of one-tenth of a point can result in intense physical changes, such as rapid heart rate, fainting, anxiety, and panic. If blood pH moves much below 6.8

or above 7.8, cells stop functioning and the patient dies. That's a shift of only six-tenths from the ideal.

Clearly, our lives "hang in the balance." No wonder the Greek philosopher Aristotle, the famed physician Galen, and the Jewish rabbi and physician Maimonides all recognized that balance was associated with health and imbalance with illness. Although the range in body weight that can sustain life is much wider than that for pH levels in the blood, the same principle applies. Too little food can lead to malnutrition, but excess eating and body weight contributes to illness.

God created the human body with a good form in mind, one that was proportioned according to precise ratios. We know a well-proportioned body when we see one, but artists and scientists have identified the ratios that appeal aesthetically and signal physical health. Symmetrical faces attract us more than asymmetrical ones because the mind interprets symmetry as connoting a healthy organism, a potential mate who is genetically equipped to produce sturdy offspring.

Leonardo da Vinci demonstrated in his classic drawings how the human arm span and distance between body parts could be reliably measured. In a well-proportioned body, for example, the distance from the top of the head to the navel holds a constant ratio to the distance from the navel to the feet. And modern science has shown that if the hip-to-waist ratio exceeds a certain point, the person has a substantially higher likelihood of heart attack. (You can guess whether it is the hip or the waist that should be the smaller number).

So when God created each of our souls and placed it in a human form, He fashioned us with love and careful attention to balance, proportion, and harmony. Through human error we often block out God's mind and fail to let it flow freely into us. If God's way is the middle path, then most extremes in life represent a deviation from God's intention. God did not create a person to be either overweight or underweight, but to maintain a healthy balance. Excess or deficient weight constitutes an imbalance that ravages bodily health.

Tikkun is the Hebrew term for healing. Restoring the body to its original, well-balanced state is an act of healing, both spiritually and physically. The body and soul become united as they were intended to be. It is one important way you can contribute to healing the microcosm of your self and bringing it into alignment with the macrocosm of the universe.

We have seen how the roots of Holy Eating can be traced back to the creation of the universe itself and the very first event in human history, eating from the tree of knowledge. Let's now turn to the ultimate source of truth, the Bible, to deepen our understanding of God's thoughts on eating.

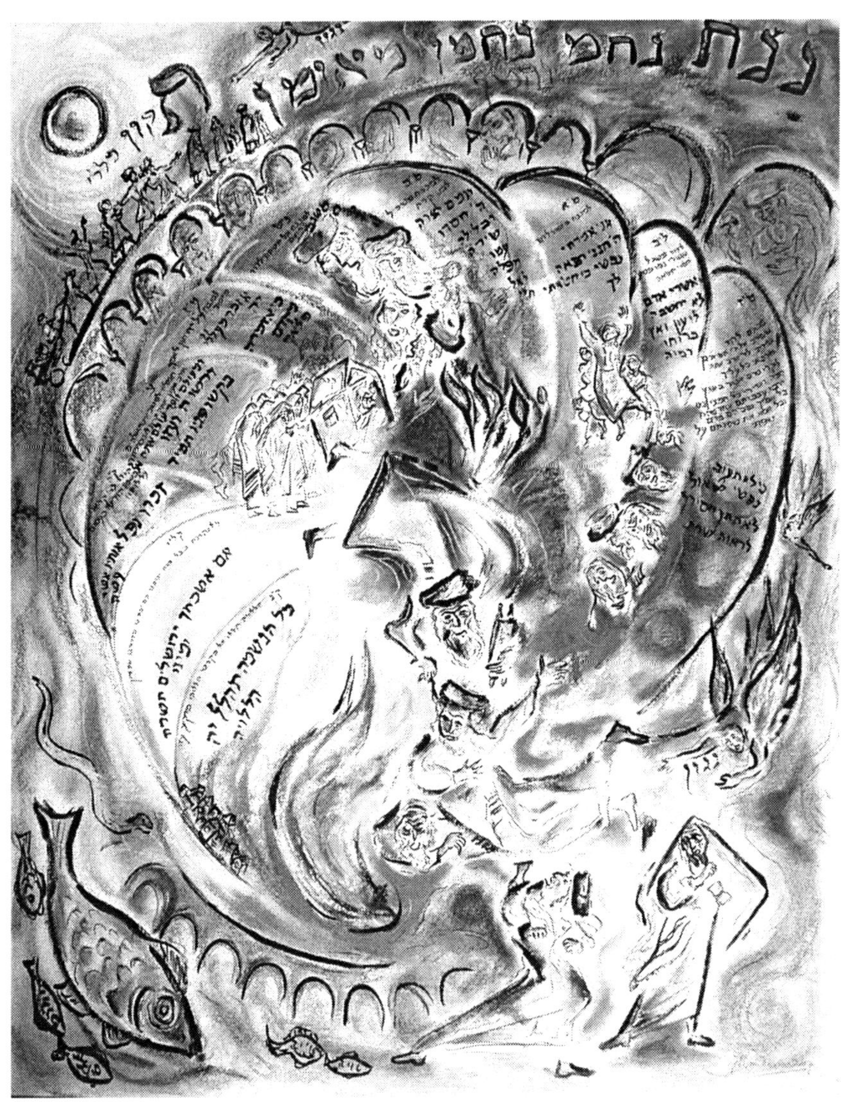

UNIVERSAL HEALING (TIKKUN KELALI)

PART II:
Does God Really Care About How I Eat?

Chapter 3

♦ ♦ ♦ ♦ ♦ ♦ ♦ ♦ ♦ ♦ ♦ ♦ ♦ ♦ ♦

The Bible: God, Humans and Food

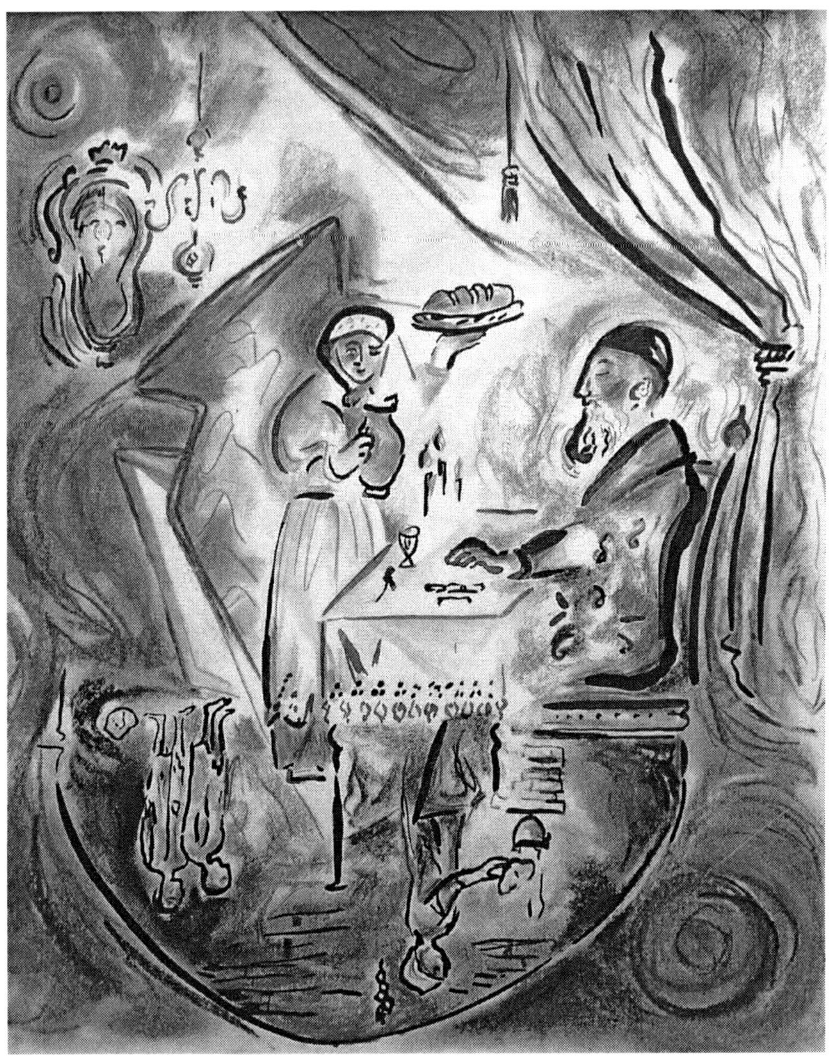

Eating Stones

> Rabbi Israel, famed Maggid (Preacher), scolded a rich ascetic who ate only a daily meal of bread and water, telling him to eat meat and other delicacies: "If the rich man dines on meat and wine, then he would at least feel that the paupers in his town should be given bread and salt. But if he himself subsists on dry bread and salt, he might think that poor people could live on stones..."

Chapters 1 and 2 provided a glimpse into the Bible's emphasis on health and proper eating. Kabbalah teaches that for an idea to be powerful enough to change behavior, it must progress beyond this initial insight and be developed in rich detail. Otherwise it remains a flash in the mind that doesn't find expression in the physical world—not a desirable outcome for weight loss! This chapter penetrates into biblical sources to expand and vitalize the idea of holy eating, so it can come alive as a compelling and irresistible truth.

What exactly does the Bible tell us about eating? Clearly, biblical law addresses what to eat, prohibiting entire categories of food, such as shellfish, and, according to rabbinic interpretation, limiting mixing meat and dairy. On fast days there's no eating or drinking for twenty-five hours, from sundown to sunset. Most major religions from Buddhism to Christianity restrict eating certain foods or declare fasts on holy days and in festival seasons.

But what does the Bible tell us about *how* to eat? The next stage of our journey will take us through biblical ideas about God, creation, food, sensuality, gluttony, health, death, sanctity, and celebration—dramatic topics on the cutting edge of life and death.

Let Us Make Man in Our Image

> *"And God said, 'Let us make Man in Our image, after Our likeness. They shall rule over the fish of the sea, the birds of the sky and over the animals, the whole earth, and every creeping thing that creeps upon the earth.' So God created Man in His image, in the image of God He created him; male and female He created them."*
>
> —*Genesis 1:26-27*

We can learn life lessons from the Biblical story of our origins: God created Man and Woman with special attention. In creating all other creatures, God used a less direct method of formation, saying, "Let the earth bring forth;" in contrast, Man[8] was created with God's more direct and personal involvement:

"Let us *make* Man"...Although every creation is imbued with God's intelligence, man is imbued with another level of Divine Providence. God created man in His image; that is to say with intellect and understanding. This concept is repeated both in this verse and later: "So God created man in His image, in the image of God He created him." When the Bible repeats something, it indicates that the concept has special importance.

Humans share with God a similar, albeit incomparable in magnitude, capacity for intelligence and understanding. Thus they are given the role of ruling over the earth and its creatures as well as freedom of choice with its attendant responsibility to make proper choices. Since man is destined to rule over the animals and the entire earth, surely he has the potential to use his intelligence and understanding to rule over himself, including how he eats. Implicit from the beginning of creation is man's capacity for ruling over himself, for self-control of his impulses, urges and wishes.

Reflection

Imagine God creating YOU in His image. That's an amazing thought. Open yourself to receive from His Divine Mind the capacity of intelligent choice and self-control of your desires. As God is Master of the Universe, you are imbued with the potential for self-mastery.

God, Physical Desires and Food

"God blessed them and God said to them, 'Be fruitful and multiply, fill the earth and subdue it; and rule over the fish of the sea, the bird of the sky, and every living thing that moves on the earth."
—Genesis 1:28

The first commandment to humankind is to be fruitful, followed by the reminder that humans must rule over every living thing, including as noted, over our selves. The second instruction to humankind is God's originally prescribed diet: "God said, 'Lo, I have given you every seed-bearing plant on the surface of the entire earth and every tree that has seed-bearing fruit; it shall be yours for food'... God saw the whole of what He had created and lo! It was very good."[9]

Note that it is only after humankind sunk into depravity and had to be regenerated through the great flood in the days of Noah that God also allowed humans to eat the flesh of animals, but with a restriction: "Every moving thing that lives shall be food for you; like the green herbage I have given you everything. But flesh, with its soul its blood you shall not eat."[10]

Thus, God's diet for humankind was originally vegetarian. But because human appetites craved animal flesh, we were later given freer range to eat of all living things, *but with restrictions.* Thus, after the flood, God's diet for man was more inclusive but not entirely free, leaving man to use his intelligence and wisdom to guide his eating and satisfy his desires for meat.

From this we learn that procreation and eating are the two essential behaviors that first occupy God's concern in guiding humankind. Created in God's image, humans must rule over nature and by extension over themselves. Appetite is naturally regulated in animals, but desire must be brought under dominion by humans, to be subdued and ruled by their intelligence. We can, in principle, control how we conduct our physical impulses and the earliest, primordial lesson in life begins with mastery over eating.

A noted 16th century Kabbalist[11] learned these core biblical truths when he was blessed for his marriage: "When I left my teacher to enter marriage, I said to him, 'Teacher! Bless me!' He answered, 'Sanctify yourself in the holiness of these two things, in eating and in intercourse. For all other mitzvahs [commandments or holy practices] do not make an impression on the body, but food sustains the body and intercourse begets the body.'"[12] Eating represents one of the primordial battlegrounds in humanity's struggle to ascend towards spiritually.

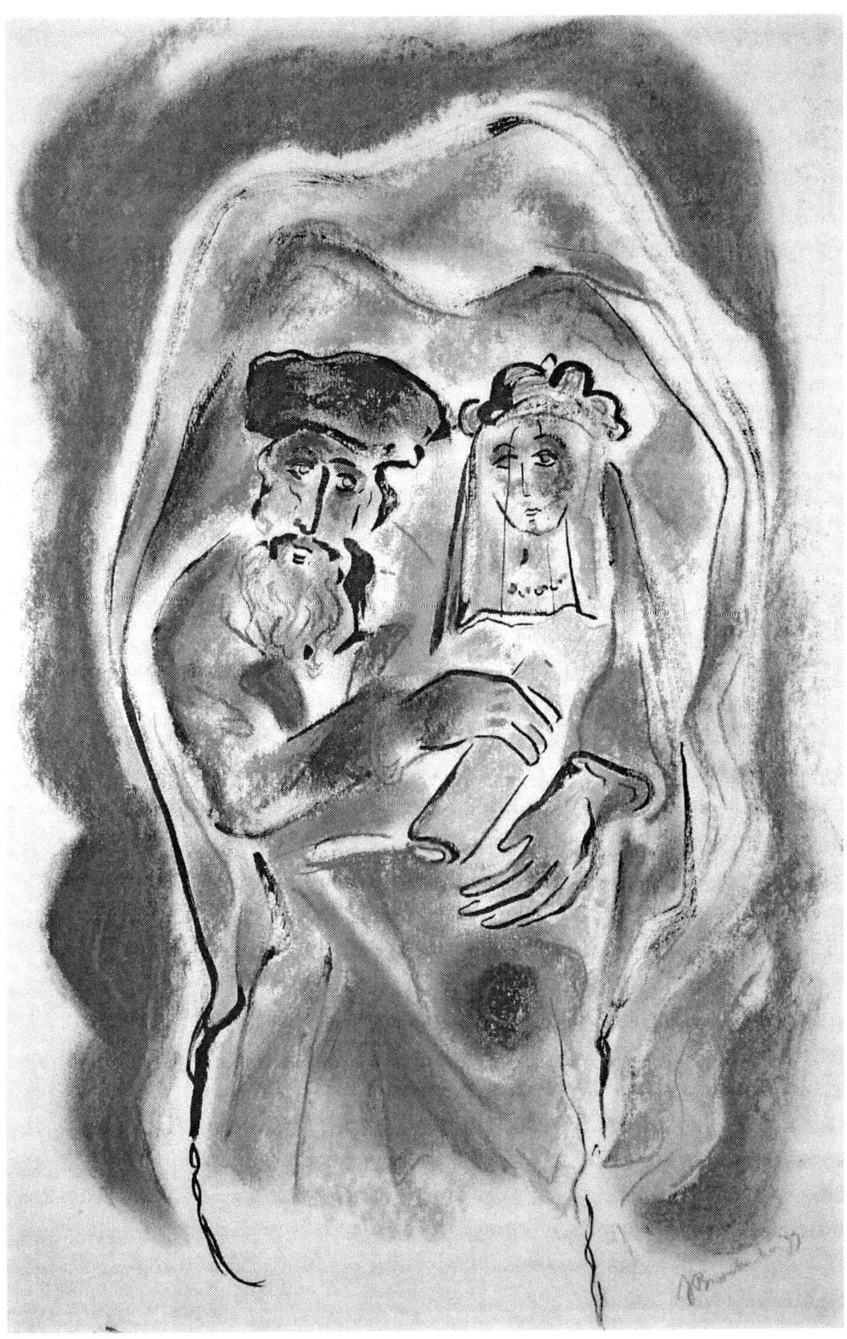

AND JACOB WEDDED RACHEL

Reflection

Ask yourself: Do I firmly believe that my intellect can rule over my behaviors and appetites? Do I think enough in constructive ways about my eating? Are my thoughts about food holy and healthy? What new thought can elevate my eating?

The Vice of Gluttony

"Stolen waters are sweet, and bread [eaten] in secret places is pleasing. But he does not know that dead men are there, that those she [the seductress] invites are in the deepest grave."
—Proverbs 9:17-18

When discussing excess eating, it is only recently that people have resumed referring to the vice of gluttony. In *The Seven Deadly Sins*, Professor Solomon Schimmel reminds us that the much ignored traditional vices—lust, greed, envy, anger, pride, sloth and gluttony—underlie most of our struggles in the pursuit of happiness and moral behavior. In addition to Adam and Eve's improper eating, the message about the dangers of gluttony was brought out early in the biblical story of Isaac's sons, Jacob and Esau: "Jacob simmered a stew, and Esau came in from the field, and he was exhausted. Esau said to Jacob, 'Pour into me, now, some of that very red stuff for I am exhausted.'"[13]

Rabbi Elie Munk, the noted French biblical scholar, observed that when Abraham's servant, Eliezer, was eating after his journey to find a wife for Abraham's son, Isaac, he said, "Let me sip." In contrast, the gluttonous and voracious Esau used the phrase "pour into me." Note also that Esau, who had a reddish complexion at birth, focuses specifically on the redness of the stew, red being the color of blood and associated with passion and lust. He also moves towards extremes, asking crudely for the *"very"* red stuff and stating not that he is merely "tired" from a day's labor, but the more extreme, *"exhausted."* He lacked balance and integration in his behavior generally and in his eating specifically.

Esau does not follow the middle path of moderation, but goes to the extreme, embodying the vice of gluttony. Gluttony, the practice of eating and drinking to excess, has dire consequences in this story and to the current day.

The consequence of Esau's excess food lust is that he sells his birthright as firstborn, his precious legacy, to his more temperate brother, Jacob, to acquire a single meal of "the very red stuff." Both Eliezer and the more refined and studious Jacob exemplify balance, moderation and self-control—essential attributes of holiness and Holy Eating.

During the wanderings in the desert, the Israelites complained about longing for the foods they savored while enslaved in Egypt:

> "But the rabble whom they had taken up into their midst had worked themselves into a lust and then the sons of Israel, too, began to weep again and said: 'Would that someone gave us meat to eat! We still remember the fish we used to eat in Egypt at no cost; the cucumbers and the melons, the leeks and the onions and the garlic, and now *our soul is dried out* [italics added], without anything; we have nothing except this *manna* before our eyes.'"[14]

Even though the manna had the luster of crystal and tasted like the delicacy of oil cakes or took on whatever taste the person desired, the people wept. Interestingly, the people do not complain about physical hunger or thirst because this was satisfied, but that their *souls* were dried out. The Bible repeatedly makes a direct linkage between eating and spirituality, between improper eating as spiritual deprivation rather than physical hunger. "Both hungry and thirsty, their soul languished within them... for He has satiated a thirsting soul, and filled a hungry soul with goodness."[15]

The Bible instructs through negative commandments as well as positive ones. Although blessings from God outweigh curses, improper behavior is not without its punishing consequences. Moses could not bear the weeping and prays to God to provide meat. God responds that they will have meat not for one day, two, five, ten or twenty days, but "for a full month until it comes out of your nostrils and will make you nauseated, because you have rejected God who is in your midst, and you have wept before Him, saying, 'Why did we leave Egypt?'"[16] The people will eat meat, but will be sickened physically because their lust represented a disconnection from God. Then God caused a wind to blow quail from the sea that piled them high throughout the camp and the Israelites spent two days and a night gathering and consuming them. "The meat was still between their teeth, nor yet chewed, when the wrath of God flared against the people, and God struck a very mighty blow [severe plague] against the people. He named that place Graves of Lust[17], because there they buried the people who had been craving."[18] God provides the requested food, but punishes with death those that overvalue the physical and reject Him by eating gluttonously.

The vice of gluttony is so central to spiritual life that it figures in Moses' summary and parting song to the Israelites as he prepares for his death:

> "Then Yeshurun [Israel] became fat and kicked—
> Whenever you became fat, you became obese and
> Overwhelmed by fat—
> And he [Israel] forsook God who had made him,
> And regarded as worthless the Rock of his salvation."[19]

Yeshurun is derived from the Hebrew word *yesher* which means straight or upright, and is used when Israel is reminded specifically to be true to its calling for moral virtue. Rabbi Samson Raphael Hirsch, the 19th century biblical commentator, noted that achieving this moral plane does not require the renunciation of earthly delights. In fact, human life can reach its pinnacle when earthly resources and pleasures are transformed into spiritual accomplishments.

Unfortunately, despite God's lessons about lust throughout the Bible and Moses' warning here, when Israel achieved material riches and pleasures, when it came out of the wilderness into a land of milk and honey, it "became fat and kicked." According to Rabbi Hirsch, this became the sadly familiar pattern of Jewish history, that Israel proved itself splendid during times of suffering, but grew obese and overgrown with fat during times of good fortune. Because of the importance of this message, I quote Rabbi Hirsch's conclusion at length:

> "The more substantial and fatty the food one introduces into the body, the more the body should seek to transform the surplus of nourishment into energy and work. The better nourished his body, the more active should the person be; the greater should be his output of activity and performance. In that case he will have control over his opulence; he will remain healthy in both mind and body; and his moral worth, too, will increase because of his greater moral and spiritual performance. But if he does not act in this manner, the surplus will be deposited in his body; he will become corpulent, obese and, instead of remaining in control over his substance, he—his true spiritual active self—will be overwhelmed by the fat, and that will be his downfall. Such has been the history of the people of Israel. It failed to utilize its abundance and surplus for increased spiritual and

> moral performance, for a more complete discharge of its task... Instead it allowed itself to become overwhelmed by wealth and prosperity, and it allowed its better spiritual, moral self to be drowned in them."[20]

This commentary, written 150 years before the advent of fast food and rampant obesity, has an amazingly modern ring. It indicates the dire consequences that we face in the current era when this ever-present problem has reached epidemic proportions.

Reflection

Imagine that YOU are facing the dramatic challenges of your Biblical ancestors: You can choose today to follow the glutton, Esau, who "poured" the food in. Or you can emulate the gourmet, Eliezer, who delicately "sipped". We have an Esau within who drives us to grow fat and kick. But all have an Eliezer waiting to emerge. Imagine the hidden Eliezer coming alive within you and personally guiding you to a more refined and Holy Eating.

Lessons from the Desert

The miraculous plagues in Egypt finally softened Pharaoh's heart and the Israelites appeared headed for freedom. But Pharaoh once again reneges and pursues them, trapping them at the edge of the Sea of Reeds. God provides the culminating miracle of splitting the sea so the Israelites can escape after which they sing the triumphant song: "God is my victory and my song; this was my salvation. This is my God and I will build Him a sanctuary...Who is like you, mighty in holiness, too awesome for praise, Doer of wonders!"[21]

Immediately after the celebration and affirmation of God's wondrous power, the people's faith is tested. As you might predict, the test relates once again to the foundation of the spiritual journey: how will His people conduct themselves in matters of eating? The Israelites wander in the Wilderness for three days and when they find water at Marah, which means "bitter", they cannot drink it because of its sharp taste. God shows Moses a tree that when thrown into the water, sweetens it and increases its volume. The people drink and are satisfied.

They arrive and set up camp at Elim where there are twelve springs of natural water and seventy date palms. As soon as they depart from the oasis of Elim, they forget the earlier bounty and God's consistent provision for their needs. They once again complain, this time more bitterly: "If only we had died by the hand of God in the land of Egypt, as we sat by the pot of meat, when we ate bread to satiety, for you have taken us out to this Wilderness to kill this entire congregation by famine."[22]

God replies to Moses: "Behold—I shall rain down for you food from heaven; let the people go out and pick each day's portion on its day, so that I can test them, whether they will follow My teaching or not."[23] The people were instructed to collect only what they needed for that day with the exception of collecting a double portion before the Sabbath because food couldn't be collected on the day of rest. On the weekdays, any food left overnight rotted, but the food left overnight for the Sabbath did not. Some of the people disobeyed God and left food overnight and it rotted. Some went to look for food on the Sabbath, but they found none.

We see again a thread of continuity where God uses food to test the spiritual mettle of the people—a trial by food rather than fire. God established the first test of eating in the Garden of Eden and now again challenges the entire people to see how they will eat on their journey to become a holy nation. A spiritual people, a nation of priests, must not rely on their own powers, but must place their faith in God. God wanted to see if their faith was strong enough to believe, as they had already witnessed, that God would prepare a table for them in the desert. As a wise sage[24] observed, one who has enough to eat today and yet worries about what they will have tomorrow must be counted among those of little faith.

This struggle continues today and God tests us daily. The difference is that today we go beyond merely worrying about tomorrow's provisions and storing up extra food for the next day. Today we eat the next day's portion at one meal! Our craving for food today is the moral equivalent of yearning for the meat pots of Egypt. Our wish to eat to satiety harkens back to the time of enslavement when the Egyptians fed us fully only to keep us strong to do hard labor the next day. Our overeating at meals is tantamount to our ancestors collecting more food than needed and saving it overnight until it became infested with worms and stank. God continues to put our spirituality to the test at each daily meal and we too often repeat the failure of our forefathers and mothers. As our Sages said: "The provision of one's daily bread is as difficult as the splitting of the Sea of Reeds."[25]

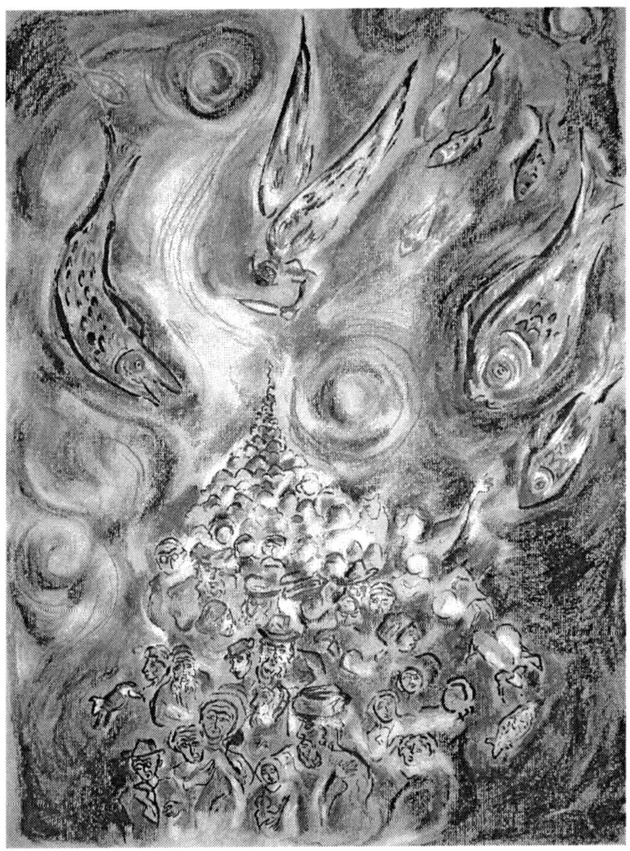

THE PARTING OF THE SEA

Reflection

While shopping for your "daily bread" or preparing the evening meal, remember the futile cravings of the Israelites who gathered excess food that became infested. Ask God to guide you to the proper foods and portion sizes. Remember that each meal is a test and each act of holy eating is a chance to affirm your faith.

Mt. Sinai and How to Eat

The Bible notes the curious but telling fact that at the highest spiritual moment of seeing the vision of God, the seventy elders, except for Moses, ate and drank:

> "Moses, Aaron, Nadab and Abihu, and seventy of the elders of Israel ascended. They saw the God of Israel, and under His feet was the likeness of sapphire brickwork, and it was like the essence of the heaven in purity. Against the great men of the Children of Israel, He did not stretch out His hand—they gazed at God, and they ate and drank."[26]

According to the several traditional commentators,[27] the onlookers sinned by irreverently indulging in food while gazing at the vision of God. Their sin was so severe that they deserved to be put to death immediately, but God did not "stretch out his Hand" to harm them so as not to diminish the joy of the moment. According to this interpretation, improper eating is once again the defining sin of even the most notable Israelites.

However, the Kabbalah offers a more mystical interpretation of the above passage that asserts the Elders did nothing wrong.[28] To the contrary, through the proper enjoyment of eating and drinking they were uplifted towards God. By eating with spiritual concentration, by Holy Eating, Man can ascend higher in spiritual elevation. Before receiving the Torah, there was a separation between the physical and spiritual, so eating at this transcendent moment could have caused God to stretch His Hand against them. But because the physical could now be permeated with spiritual energy, it was fitting to eat while gazing at God—as long as it was done with holiness. This feast was a meritorious act of rejoicing in the gift of the Torah, the five books of Moses, and the prototype event for uplifting the physical and enjoying meals at holy occasions.

Celebrating God's wonders with holy feasts has such a strong tradition that it inspired the quip about Jewish history boiling down to a simple formula: "They tried to kill us, we won, let's eat." But sadly, many carry this to the unholy extreme of excess eating with untoward consequences. In fact, this may go a long way towards explaining the seeming paradox that some otherwise spiritual people today are overweight: Their very spiritual nature strongly impels them towards the celebratory use of food, but they have disconnected from spiritual concentration at the times of meals. Reconnecting those strong spiritual wires to the act of eating can result in a rapid transformation for such persons.

Both of the above views illustrate that eating, if done properly can be elevating, but if done in prohibited or extreme ways can bring devastating consequences, even death. The linkage of receiving the Torah with eating at first seemed curious, but is consistent with our view that it is at the heart of spirituality. Recall that the first event in the life of humankind was the prohibited eating by Adam and Eve.

We are taught that when two opinions of the sages seem to contradict each other, they both contain truth that can be reconciled at another level of understanding. If this act of eating was irreverent, it could bring death as we see today that gluttonous eating may bring death; if the eating was acceptable, then it was done as an offering to God as a way of elevating oneself through Holy Eating at the most sublime moment of spiritual connection. The message is clear: Food and spirituality are inextricably linked, but how one eats can either elevate or degrade. Unholy eating can cause death, but Holy Eating preserves life and can be a springboard to eternal weight transformation.

Reflection

Prepare for your next religious holiday or joyous occasion now. You can be certain there will be food. Remind yourself that the Elders ate after receiving the Torah, but they ate with holiness. Remember that the primary reason you are there is to celebrate, not to eat. Focus on the spiritual meaning of the holiday or the joy of the wedding occasion rather than the food itself.

The Essential Torah of Eating

The universal truth contained in ancient wisdom speaks to our most modern struggles. Pleasure has a place in spiritual life, but we are instructed to shift from our personal pleasure alone to the greater pleasure of loving and serving God. The Code of Jewish Law advises:

> "For everything from which you derive benefit or enjoyment in this world, your intention should be not your own pleasure but to serve God, blessed be He, as it is written, 'Know Him

in all your ways.' Our Sages said, 'Let all your deeds be for the sake of heaven.' Even things of personal choice, such as eating and drinking, walking, sitting and standing, conversation, and everything connected with the needs of your body—all should be for the service of God, or for something that leads to the service of God. So even if you are hungry and thirsty, if you ate and drank for your own pleasure it is not praiseworthy; you should intend that you are eating and drinking to keep yourself alive for the service of God."[29]

Maimonides, or Rambam, the 13th century rabbi and physician to the Sultan of Egypt, brings the healer's eye to detect the importance of these laws for bodily health:

"A man should direct his mind and all his actions exclusively to knowing God. Whether sitting, rising, or talking—all must be bent in this direction...Also, when he eats and drinks and has relations he should not do this only to gratify his physical needs, so that he is likely to eat and drink only what is sweet to the palate and have relations only for pleasure, but should have in mind that he eats and drinks for the sole purpose of maintaining his body and its organs in good health. Hence he will not eat everything that the palate desires, like a dog or a donkey, but will use foods which do good to the body, whether bitter or sweet, avoiding those that are harmful to the body even though they are sweet to the palate."[30]

These are very strong words if we pause to read them carefully and carry them to their logical conclusion. The Talmud is equally explicit about not eating as an animal does: "Our sages taught: One who eats in the street is comparable to a dog. There are those who say that he is disqualified from serving as a witness."[31] Essentially, Maimonides, supported by the sages, is instructing us to act as a human being, not a dog or a donkey that consumes everything it desires. Proper eating is a choice, not merely how to consume food, but whether to act as a person or an animal. Recall the earlier distinction between eating with God-consciousness rather than self-consciousness that underlies Holy Eating.

Maimonides clearly states that it is a duty to cultivate health and avoid what is harmful to the body because this enables us to have the strength to serve God better. By keeping the body in good health one follows the ways of God because it is impossible to understand or serve the Creator when one is ill. So it is our duty to shun whatever is harmful to the body and cultivate health-preserving habits. The formula is simple: *A man should not eat except when he is hungry, nor drink except when he is thirsty.*[32]

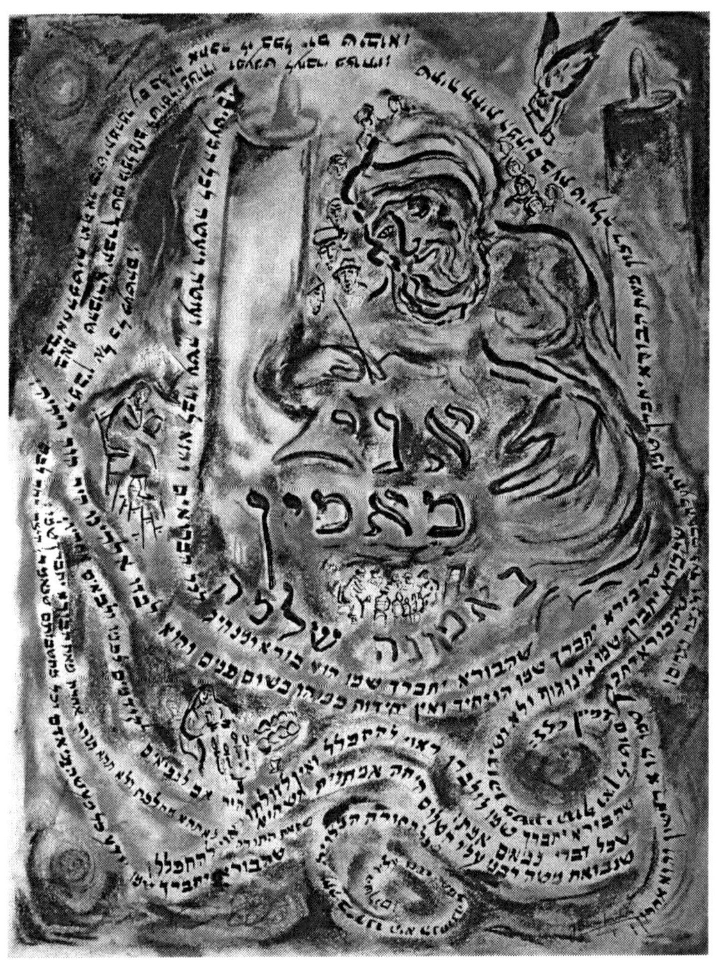

The Principles of Maimonides (Rambam)

Not only should people eat or drink only when hungry, they should not fully satiate themselves when eating: "He should not eat until his stomach is full. Rather he should stop before his appetite is fully satisfied, using one-fourth less food than would completely gratify him."[33] This prescription is echoed in Proverbs (13:25): "The righteous eats to appease his soul, but the stomach of the wicked is never satisfied." Research conducted at the University of Wisconsin National Primate Center supports this ancient wisdom. Monkeys that have been maintained for 17 years on a high nutrition but calorie restricted diet live longer, look younger, are more youthful and energetic, and develop fewer or no diseases at all. Calorie intake was reduced by 30%, almost exactly the amount recommended by Maimonides over 900 years ago.

If we take these words seriously, the inescapable conclusions may seem harsh. But given Maimonides' authoritative voice, let's be clear about his meaning: The "righteous" person who "follows the ways of God," eats only when hungry and what is needed for sustenance. The person who eats even when not hungry, who eats more than what is needed for sustenance, is not following the way of God in this respect and is not acting righteously. We are in effect commanded to eat in the style of Jacob and Eliezer, not as Esau. Excessive overeating is clearly defined as improper eating and is thus a sin that distances us from God.[34]

The biblical message that we must eat healthful foods sparingly and only when hungry is consistent with the profound words of Rabbi Shneur Zalman of Liadi, the Alter Rebbe[35], 18th century originator of the Chabad movement who first brought the wisdom of the Kabbalah to a wider audience: *"What is forbidden is forbidden and what is permitted is not necessary."* Certain foods are forbidden and must not be eaten; but simply because healthful and permitted foods are more than ever in abundant supply, there is no necessity to consume them. Imagine how cutting your consumption of food by 25% will affect your weight.

Reflection

Memorize and contemplate daily the Alter Rebbe's maxim: "What is forbidden is forbidden and what is permitted is not necessary." His follower who heard these words said that for three or four years we labored over them until the knowledge was integrated into our lives. Only then would we go for our first private meeting with the Rebbe. Think deeply about why you take more than you need and ask yourself before indulging: "Do I really need this?" "Even if it's permitted, is it necessary?" Remind yourself and meditate upon this daily.

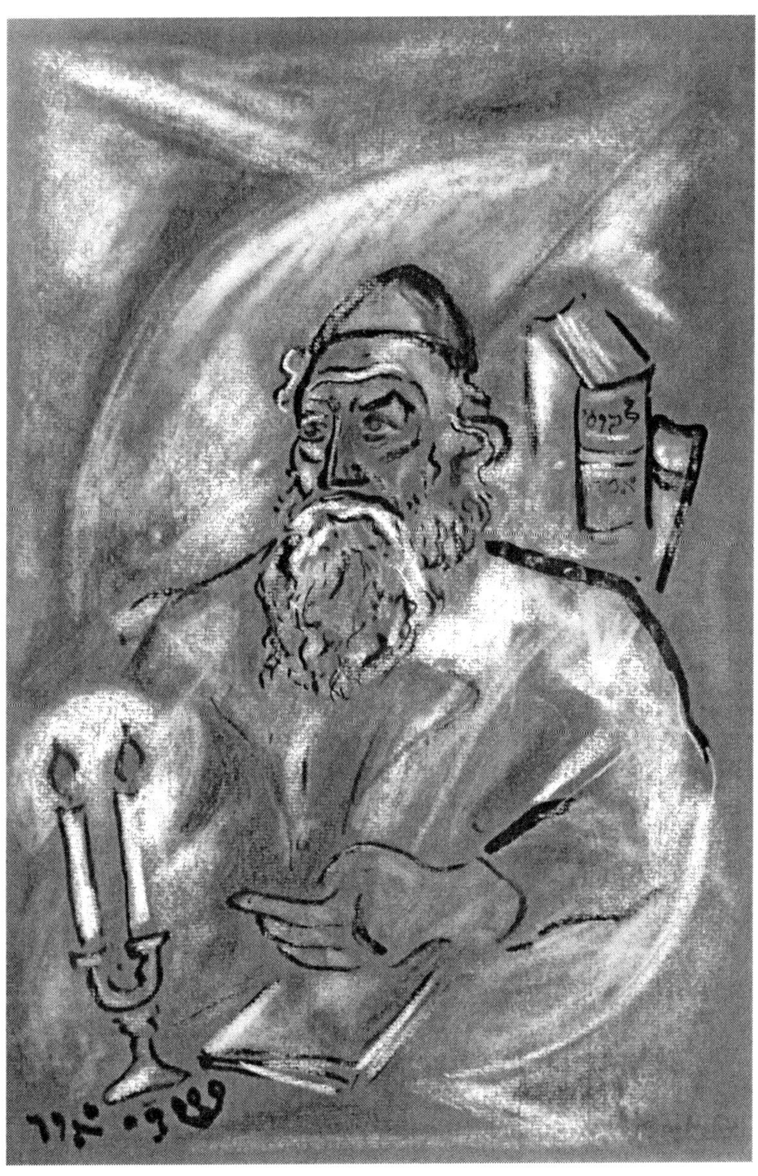

RABBI SHNEUR ZALMAN OF LIADI (THE ALTER REBBE)

Wisdom of the Body in Prayer

Since the first major events in human history recorded in the Bible involved the physical act of eating, we should not be surprised that one of the first morning prayers said daily after washing the hands, is about bodily functioning:

> "Blessed are You, Lord our God, King of the universe, who has formed man in wisdom, and created within him numerous orifices and cavities. It is revealed and known before the Throne of Your Glory that if but one of them were to be blocked, or one of them were to be opened, it would be impossible to exist even for a short while. Blessed are You, Lord, who heals all flesh and performs wonders."[36]

The day begins, not with attention to the spirit or soul, but with a focus on the body that is the foundation of our existence in life. The prayer that follows this one–"My God, the soul which You have given within me is pure…"– thanks God for giving us a soul and restoring it to us in the morning after sleep. Bodily function is attended to first and then the soul, not the other way around. This is not to say that the body is more important than the soul. But since the body is the dwelling place of the soul, we must first express gratitude for the marvels of its physical function. Human life begins with the physical and ascends toward the spiritual.

The idea that the physical is a dwelling place for spiritual forces captures what may be the core concept of Kabbalah, as we will see in the next chapter.

Chapter 4

◆ ◆

The Kabbalah of Eating

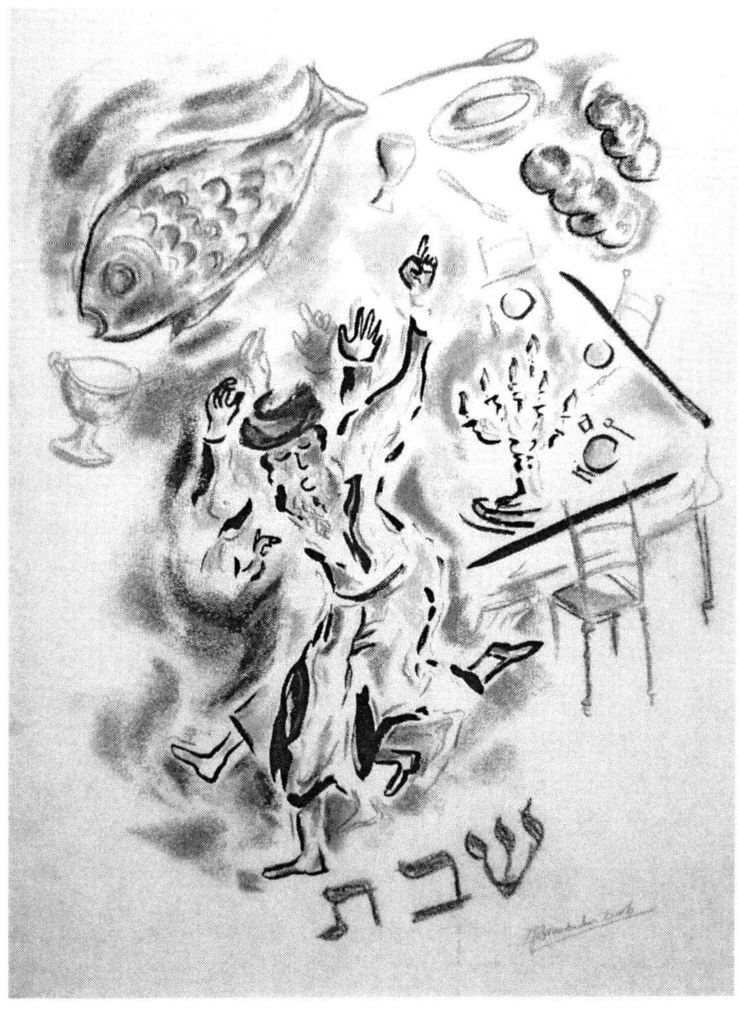

The Table

The Baal Shem Tov spent the Sabbath in Kolomaya where he sensed the presence of a holy soul radiating great light. So he went for a stroll and saw the light radiating from a certain home where he heard the sounds of singing and dancing. Seeing that the door was slightly ajar, he went in and saw Rabbi Yaakov Koppel dancing in ecstasy before his Shabbat table, which was laden with good food. Rabbi Koppel sang and danced for a long time before noticing the Baal Shem Tov. He welcomed his guest warmly, and the Besht asked him,

"Why do you sing and dance this way before eating?"

Rabbi Yaakov Koppel answered,

"Before I partake of the physical food, I first stand in front of the table and absorb the food's spiritual essence. Sometimes I become so aroused that I sing and dance."

What is the food's "spiritual essence"? It is its divine aspect. A Jewish mystic meditates on how the food has been created and is being kept in existence (like all created things) every minute by God's will. And a person's profound realization that God has created this food to nourish and provide for him leads him to mystic joy.

Excerpted by permission from Jewish Tales of Mystic Joy by Yitzhak Buxbaum, JosseyBass, 2002.

The Kabbalah teaches that spirituality should not be relegated exclusively to abstract higher spheres of existence. Spiritual principles need to become tangible and apparent in a person's flesh and blood. We must not abandon physicality in search of spirituality. Our goal is to make the physical world sensitive and receptive to the Divine. The term Kabbalah means to "receive" which implies receiving higher spiritual truths from above and making our everyday world of physicality receptive to spiritual energies. Just as hardened earth must be plowed to accept seeds, we must refine our physical selves to let God in.

Making a Home for God in the World

As we saw earlier, ancient Jewish wisdom tells us we are here to know and to serve God. Famed Kabbalist, Rabbi Isaac Luria, taught that God is purely good and God's natural desire is to bestow this goodness upon others in abundance. Goodness can be given only if there is someone to receive it, so God created the world and mankind to receive His goodness. Chassidic philosophy[37] teaches that we must first make a home for God in the material world so that God's divine presence can be fully received.

But what exactly does this mean? Isn't God everywhere and therefore already here and at home? Not necessarily. Although we don't have to bring God into the material world, He can be *in the world* without being *at home* here. The physical world is naturally egocentric with every object and animal simply existing to promote its own needs or self-preservation. People can go to great extremes to pursue self-advancement.

This selfishness is inherent in the material world, but masks the truth that creation of the world is not an end in itself but a vehicle of the Creator to bestow goodness. To make our world a home for God, we must therefore *transform* its very nature from something that exists for itself into something that exists for a purpose greater than itself, to serve God, to know God, to receive God's goodness.

When a person takes a material object and makes it into a religious ritual object, this effects such a transformation. Money kept in the pocket indicates self-interest and greed. If one gives money to another as charity, this transforms the money into serving a higher purpose of bestowing good onto others rather than keeping it to serve oneself. Leather used to make a saddle does not reach the same level as when it is used to cover a prayer book. There are two steps in making our world a home for God: forging the material object into a vessel for Godliness and actually using the object to serve the divine will. It would seem that using the object would be more important. Yet the Bible spends more time describing the details of the construction of the Holy Temple, for example, than it does on how to implement the services to God. Why is this so?

From this we learn that the stage of *construction* is more vital than the stage of *implementation*. That is, the formative process of making ourselves into vessels to receive Godliness is more important than the final step of actually bringing Godliness into our lives. The reason is that this is where the actual point of transformation from a self-centered object into something committed to a higher purpose occurs. ***God delights especially in the creative work of self-transformation.*** Process, not perfection, should be our focus.

God could have created a purely spiritual and perfect world that would have been a more hospitable environment to receive His goodness. But He created the material, self-focused world because He desires the act of transformation itself, the transcendent process that elevates the material into the spiritual. God desires the process of struggle, growth and change that uplifts our nature so we can connect with and receive spiritual goodness.

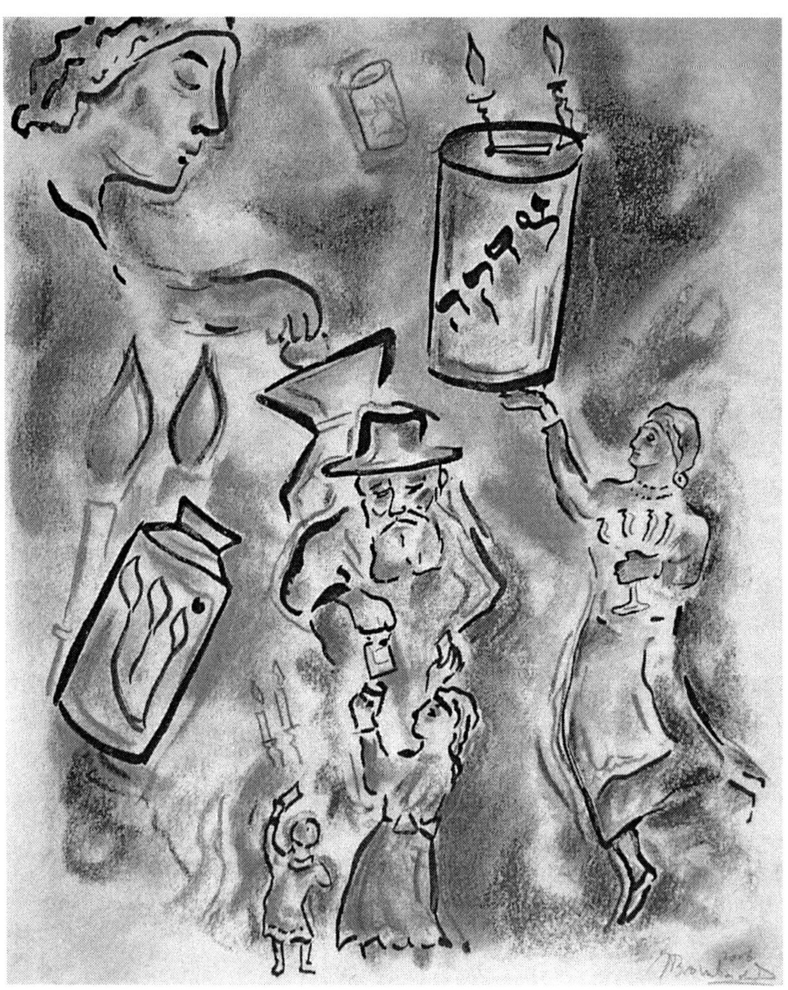

CHARITY (TZEDAKAH)

Since the soul dwells in the body, the first human challenge of self-transformation is to master and elevate our physical body. We make the body a vessel for our Godly soul, not by denying or disconnecting from it, but by recognizing its higher spiritual purpose.

The path of Kabbalah is to find the middle path, the balance between extremes of asceticism and overindulgence. When eating is self-centered and excessive, this signifies greed that is similar to keeping all of one's money rather than sharing it with others. The body is altered, but in a negative, self-destructive direction. The physical dominates and the body says, " I exist for myself and my own purpose which is to satisfy my selfish needs." The physical is not transformed, but strengthened. The results of ill health can signify the failure of self-transformation. With each act of restraint, the body says, "I exist not for myself, but for a purpose higher than myself, to become a vessel for Godliness, to serve and know God, to be strong and live a long and vigorous life so I can give to others, as God bestows goodness on me."

The Body is a Temple for the Soul

The instructions for the Holy Temple in Jerusalem were given in extraordinary detail, taking up a surprisingly large section of the Bible. Beauty and adornment were paramount concerns in addition to the holy functions to be performed there. The size, shape and proportion were designed with great precision. The Temple was the physical vessel in which God's spirit dwelled among the people: "Make for Me a Sanctuary and I will dwell amongst you." [38]

After God leads Israel triumphantly across the Sea of Reeds to safety from the pursuing Egyptians, Moses leads them in a song that includes this declaration of faith: "This is my God and I will build Him a sanctuary; the God of my father and I will exalt him."[39] However, another translation by Samson Raphael Hirsch personalizes this further: "Henceforth this will be my God; to Him would I *be a habitation*. He was already my father's God; I would raise Him higher still (italics added)." The renowned biblical commentator, Rashi, adds that the terms "raise higher" or "exalt" can also be translated as "beautify." Thus, "I will beautify Him by relating His praises."

The first translation suggests the desire to construct a building, a physical Temple, to praise and exalt God; the second, according to Hirsch, emphasizes offering one's self as a dwelling place for God: all my life and all my being shall become a personal Temple dedicated to His glorification, a place in which He will be revealed. And following Rashi, the Sages add that one should strive to serve God in a beautiful manner.

It follows that although the spiritual is of primary importance, God also wanted a physical Temple made to precise specifications for Him to dwell in. Similarly, although the transcendent soul is our higher self, the soul dwells in a corporeal body. We must serve God in a beautiful way with all of our lives and all of our being, including the body. We need to be a habitation for God and we should beautify this dwelling place both in how we conduct ourselves in all aspects of life and in how we look physically. Body and soul must be one. Ideally, the beauty of the soul will project outwardly and be expressed in the refinement of the body.

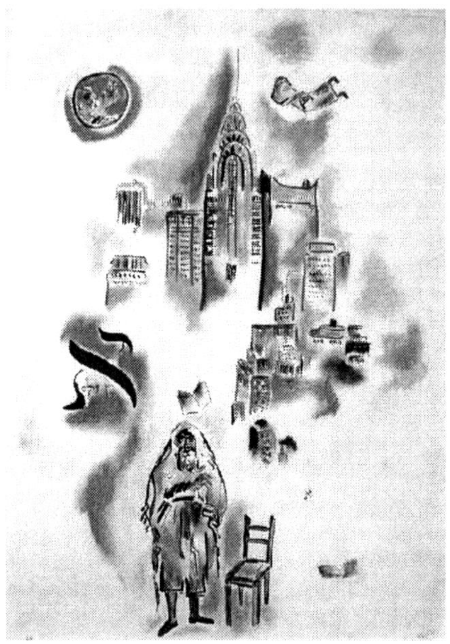

ETERNAL LORD (ADON OLAM)

In Kabbalah we learn that all creation begins with God and descends through four levels to become the physical world that we as humans know and dwell in. One of these levels is the world of *formation* where the spiritual ideas of God are shaped into physical form and given substance. Your body is one of these forms. As is descends through the levels of existence, changes can occur in its outer appearance—its garments. Through negative thoughts and behaviors, the outer garments can become distorted and out of balance, but the inner core of the spiritual essence remains pure.

So it is with excess weight. The essence of your physical form in God's mind is your optimal shape, the precise specifications by which you were made. When you lose connection to the spiritual realm, the body expresses this in weight gain and bodily distortions of the ideal form. By reconnecting with God, by returning to the heavenly source of existence, you can become one with your intended ideal form; you can unify your body with your soul; you can restore the balance and harmony that is God's intention for you. You can purify and rededicate your body, the Temple of the soul.

Elevating the Sparks in Food

According to Kabbalah, when the world was created the intensity of divine light was so powerful that the original vessels could not contain it and shattered into shards or broken fragments. Sparks of divinity fell to the lowest levels of physical existence and became hidden in husks or shells. Through our spiritual practices and quest for re-unification with God, we can discover and elevate these hidden sparks. The ultimate task of humankind is to repair the world through good deeds that release these holy sparks from their shell and unite the physical with the spiritual. Only by cracking the hard shell of a walnut do we reveal the life preserving, Omega 3 rich food hidden within.

Every physical thing contains within it the vital energy of God—the Shechinah—without which it would cease to exist. Food especially has this spiritual side that co-exists with the material side. Kabbalah teaches that eating with God-consciousness elevates the holy sparks within the food. Remember that because the food comes from God, it must be consumed in a refined, moderate and balanced way. When we eat out of desire to satisfy only physical needs, Kabbalah warns that we fail to ignite the holy sparks and instead strengthen the dark or evil side.

The Baal Shem Tov, founder of the Chassidic or Pietistic movement, suggested a higher level beyond eating properly to preserve health in order to serve God in the future. He said that in everything you do for the sake of heaven, you should see that there is some holy service of God within the act itself: "For example, in eating, do not just say that your intention in eating for the sake of heaven is so that you should have energy afterwards to serve God—although that is certainly *also* a good intention. Nevertheless, the essence of spiritual perfection will be when the deed done for the sake of heaven has an immediate connection to the service of God—such as lifting up the holy sparks within the food."[40] Eating to preserve future health is often weak motivation to resist the chocolate layer cake or chips on your plate. If you yearn to be connected to God at all times, stay in the moment and make each meal a holy service.

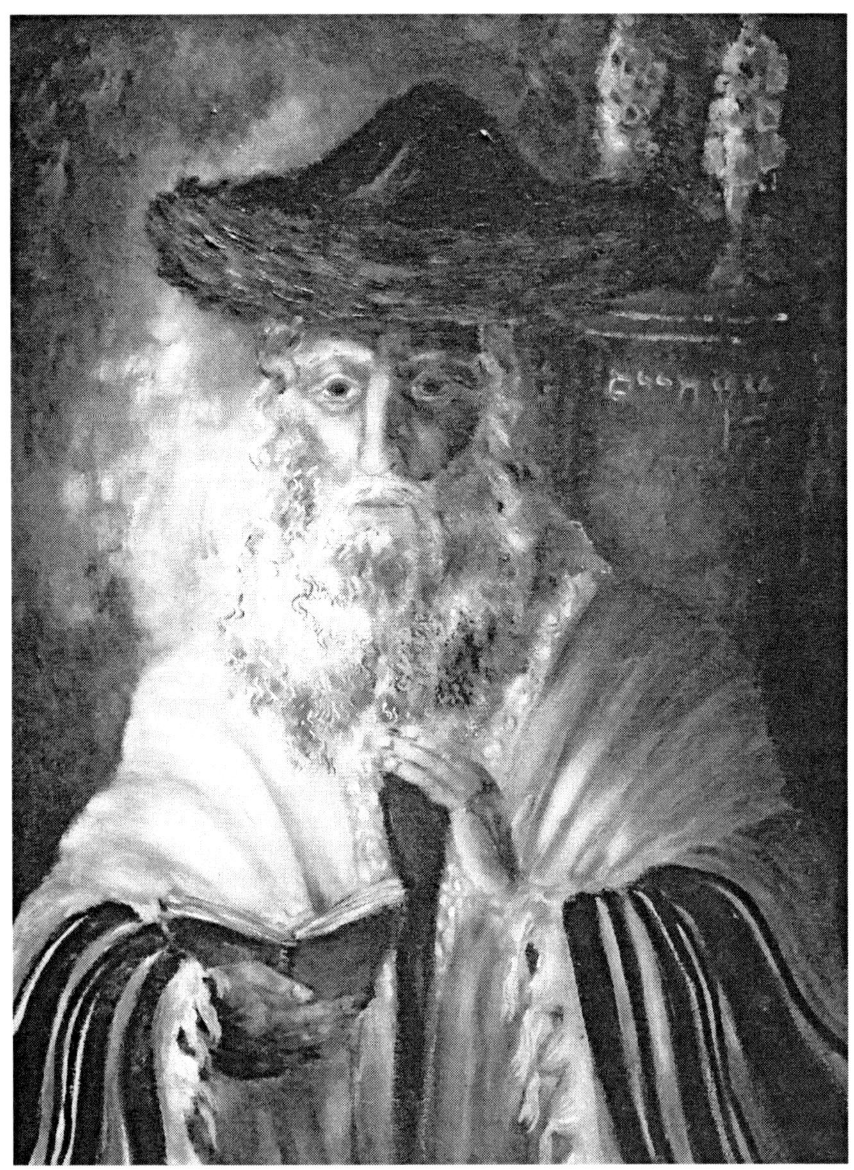

The Baal Shem Tov (The Besht)

Three Levels of Eating

Let's build on Baal Shem Tov's idea of going beyond eating to serve God to making the act of eating itself a form of service to God. We can distinguish one form of self-conscious eating (Serving Self) and two forms of God-conscious eating (Serving God and Service to God).

Level 1 Eating: Serving Self

Self-conscious eating involves eating that focuses on pleasure for the self. At worst, it is a form of lust that consumes food as a hungry animal; at best, it consumes less ravenously, but still is directed only towards bodily and sensual pleasure from the act of eating devoid of spiritual connection. This form of eating does not elevate the sparks in the food, but rather strengthens the dark or evil side that can cause imbalances that result in negative states of ill health and obesity.

Level 2 Eating: Serving God

The first level of God-conscious eating is to eat primarily, not for self-pleasure, but to sustain the self in order to be able later to serve God. One must eat healthfully to be strong and prolong life to better perform God's will. As the sages observed, men of good deeds would say before meals that they want to eat and drink so they will healthy and strong to better serve God. This level of eating does not strengthen the dark forces, but does not in itself elevate the sparks in the food. Since it is eaten with the idea of empowering oneself to better serve God in the future, it can lead to more deeds that might elevate holy sparks related to these actions, but it does not accomplish this directly.

Level 3 Eating: Service to God

The highest level of God-conscious eating is to eat, not to later be able to serve God, but to make the current act of eating itself a service to God. This highest level of eating transforms the experience of pleasure from eating into a direct connection with the holy sparks in the food. Such eating does not bring purely *sensual pleasure* derived from the body of the food, but rather yields a more *holistic, integrated joy* that is drawn from the very soul or essence of the food. As an analogy, consider how the few drops of oil derived from the essence of the olive yields fuel that provides fire and illumination. Kabbalah does not promote asceticism, but transforms and elevates sensual pleasure into holy joy that integrates and elevates. Note the connection between the terms holistic and holy.

This level of eating can lead to mystical or ecstatic states, as with a revered Sage who experienced eating as though it were from the: "Upper table that is before God, and his food is coming to him from God's hand... Such a person, although he is in this world, his mind is not here, but in the World to Come."[41] It is unlikely that every meal will be eaten at this level. Yet one can strive for at least part of each meal to bring a degree of mindful concentration that recognizes God as the bountiful source of food. Elevate the meal by expressing gratitude to God and to the many human and animal agents throughout the complex food chain who were responsible for bringing this sustenance to your holy table.

Eating as Higher Than Prayer

"Bread should be eaten on the edge of a sword."
—Zohar—

As surprising at it sounds, certain kabbalistic sages viewed the seemingly mundane act of eating as even more important spiritually than prayer itself. How can this be? A noted Chassidic mystic[42] explained:

> "Most people exert all their energy in the time of prayer, to direct their heart and to ward off foreign thoughts. But when they eat they make no effort or exertion, since they eat only for their own pleasure—so where is there a place for effort or exertion? But as the saintly persons, the tzaddikim, of blessed memory, have already said: 'The time of eating is a time of war.' The tzaddikim have no need to exert themselves when they pray; then, their minds are always pure and clear. But during the time of eating, that is when they have to use their energy and exert themselves."[43]

The time of eating is a time of war. What seems paradoxical can be easily recognized by anyone who has fought the "battle of the bulge" only to lose ground and relapse to excess eating and weight gain. If prayer comes naturally to a person, there is less need for transformation since the act comes easily to her.

We learned earlier that God desires the process of transformation and growth more than the ultimate result. Since many struggle with food craving, there is abundant opportunity for transformation in this arena. The battle over improper eating–being the first struggle in the history of humankind and the earliest in the life of each individual–is the foremost battleground for personal and spiritual development. Recall that God's first instruction to Adam and Eve was about how to eat, not about how to pray. For this reason, achieving Holy Eating can bring one to a higher level of spirituality than even prayer.

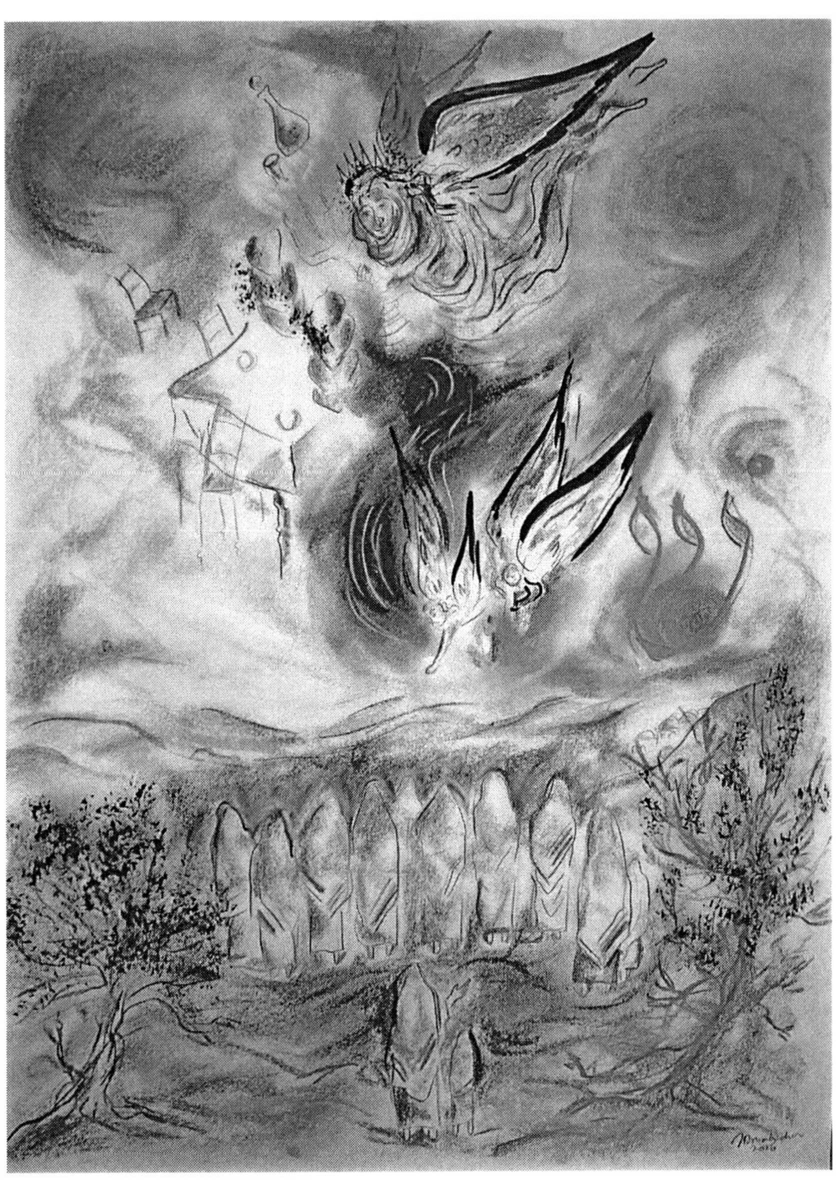

RECEIVING QUEEN SHABBAT IN TZFAT (SAFED)

PART III:
How to Make Your Meals Holy

Chapter 5

◆ ◆ ◆ ◆ ◆ ◆ ◆ ◆ ◆ ◆ ◆ ◆ ◆ ◆ ◆ ◆

The Spiritual Steps to Holy Eating

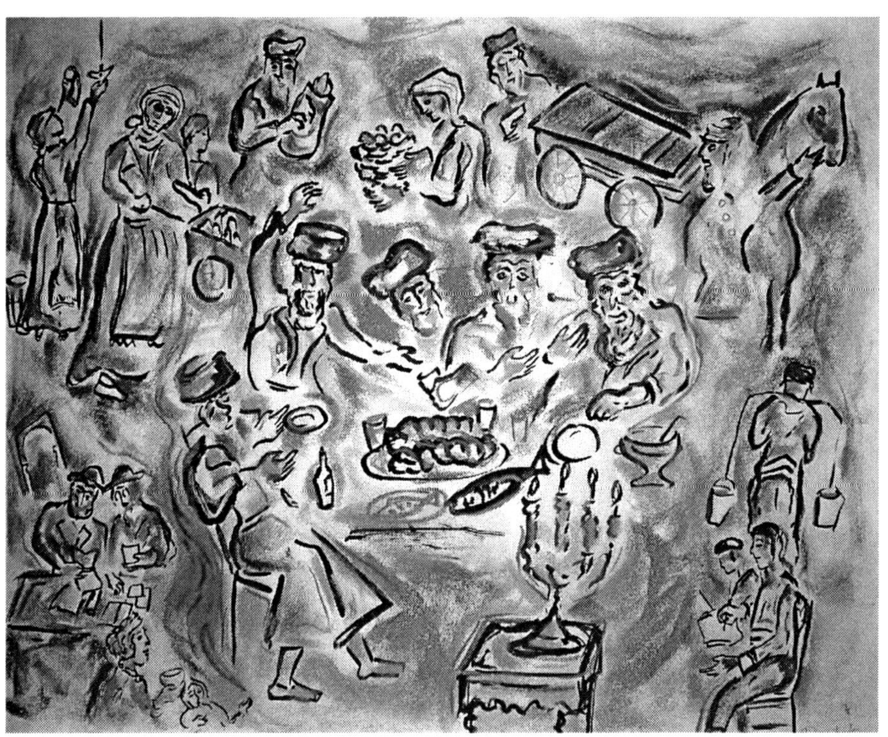

Shabbos Coats and Fur Hats (Shtraymels)

Reb Zusya and his brother Elimelech had a problem. Whenever they ate and sang together with their Chassidim on the Sabbath (Shabbos) they were overcome with holiness and enthusiasm. Their shabbos tish (table) was always intense and beautiful.

But they wondered: What caused these great feelings of joy? Was it the Sabbath itself or were they just carried away by the singing, the food, the fine sabbath clothes and the company? They decided to do an experiment to find out.

On a routine Tuesday, they prepared a wonderful sabbath meal with everything you could wish for: delicious foods, bottles of shnaps, a samovar for hot tea, and the best white tablecloth. They wore satin coats and beautiful shtraymels (fur hats) for Shabbos. Before sunset they came together with their Chassidim and the dancing was so vigorous that the walls shook, and the room seemed engulfed in a fiery radiance. The candles glowed, the wine flowed, many words of Torah were spoken and a sumptuous meal served. Outside was the hustle and bustle of a normal weekday, but inside the room it was Shabbos. The Chassidim sang so loudly that they did not hear what was going on in the busy streets of the town.

But Reb Zusya and Rebbe Elimelech couldn't accept that mere objects or songs, or even the beautiful words of Torah, caused their enthusiasm for this "Shabbos on a weekday!" They decided to make the long trip to their revered Rebbe, the Maggid of Mezeritch, who would have an answer for them. When they poured out their heart to him he smiled because he was impressed with their piety.

"Look", he said, "what is so bad if you get into a Shabbos mood when you wear your sthraymels and your nice coats on a weekday and have all your Shabbos dishes in front of you? Those objects are connected with Shabbos in your mind and they attract the spirit of Shabbos. You are, thank God, very receptive to that. And I know you both: You are very serious in your zeal to serve God, so I don't see a problem: You want to serve God and you also enjoy Shabbos, which is connected with serving God! Beautiful! I wish you a good Shabbos and many more celebrations!"

Reb Zusya and his brother Rebbe Elimelech returned home in an upbeat mood! May we all experience Shabbos as they did and celebrate every meal with holiness and joyful enthusiasm.

If you already engage in daily spiritual practices, you may now be ready to eat in a holy way. This single powerful idea—that God wants you to be holy, healthy, and trim—can generate immense energy, enough to transform your eating habits and weight permanently. But most people—particularly those who do not practice their religion daily—will need the cognitive-behavioral strategies outlined in this chapter to translate their spiritual knowledge into everyday habits. Otherwise, when faced with a favorite candy bar or overpowering midnight hunger, they may lose the battle. They may say I "know" what I should do, I "know" that I shouldn't eat so much, or even I "know" that God wants me to be different, but…

The problem is that such statements use the word "know" in its most superficial sense. To "know" can mean merely to be aware of something, or it can mean to have a thorough understanding through laborious study or life experiences. In the biblical sense, as when Adam "knew" Eve physically, two separate entities merge in the most intimate form of knowing. The Kabbalah refers to this level of knowing as *Daas*, or true knowledge that integrates the initial spark of understanding–*Chochmah*–with the detailed particulars—*Binah*.

Hearing something once, having a noble idea float into mind, or even a cursory reading of a book do not constitute "knowing" in this sense. Initial knowing often comes in a burst of enthusiasm, but, like infatuation in love, it fades at the first major obstacle. Such superficial knowing is weak tea against the temptations of food. Deep knowledge in the biblical sense comes from intense study, memorization, transforming ideas into systematic beliefs and disciplined behavioral repetition. In a religious framework, the process of developing these beliefs is referred to as **spiritual transformation**. In contemporary psychology, it's called **cognitive restructuring**—developing and adopting improved ways of thinking, weaving these into a coherent belief system, and linking these new beliefs to behaviors and feelings through repeated experience. Only this kind of deep wisdom will sustain the application of these life-altering ideas. The initial spark of excitement about taking on a religious life must be followed by intense study and practice.

The kabbalists developed spiritual practices with the aim of applying divine knowledge to daily activities, including eating. Inspired by their approach, this chapter draws upon cognitive-behavioral strategies to help integrate new thinking and eating habits into your everyday life.

The Power of Purpose

The first step in any cognitive-behavioral change program is to establish a definite sense of purpose, a strong motivational set. Consistent with kabbalistic thinking, your purpose should address both levels of existence: **the divine and the human**, the spiritual and the physical.

Divine Purpose

As we learned, Kabbalah teaches that God's divine purpose was to create a physical world. Your bodily existence is an expression of God's divine will. You might say that God had a picture of how you would look physically as well as the nature of your soul, your true inner self. Search within yourself to find your true body image, one that respects your body type. Some people will be shorter and rounder by nature, others tall and slim. But most do not find excess fat to be part of their healthy, optimal body image. Rabbi Akiva Tatz observed that beauty exists when the inner soul matches the outer physical expression. But when the outer expression fails to match the inner soul, we feel shame. When you find within yourself your true body image and bring your physical form into alignment with it, you will achieve and radiate beauty. You will have aligned yourself with God's will.

Although human and divine purpose are both important, the greatest power to change can come from knowing and embracing the divine. For those who already follow God's instructions about other aspects of life, including what to eat (e.g., fasts, kosher diet, periods of meatless meals) and when to pray, work, and rest, this step can be readily attained.

Most people simply have not connected how they eat with a clear sense that God really does care about this part of life. Something has blocked the flow of energy within them regarding this fundamental truth. Once the connection is strongly formed, desire is transformed and the struggle to control eating is eased. The goal is to progress from an abstract understanding of the idea of Holy Eating to personally believing it as true for you. **When**

you accept that God is interested in how *you* eat, your sense of purpose can explode into a fiery passion, transforming your relationship to food and to your body.

God's will is internalized, unified with your personal motivation. The energy gain will be like shifting from a conventional furnace to a nuclear energy plant. You will know how Moses and Miriam would eat and you will be able to do the same.

Have you ever fasted or given up a type of food for spiritual reasons? Perhaps you struggled or did so with ease, but either way you succeeded in completing the fast. How did you manage to do it? You had a sense of higher purpose that transcended your personal desires. You believed at some level that God wanted you to fast or deny yourself something for the prescribed period of time and you followed this instruction.

The same belief can lead you to transform your eating every day, not only on fast days. Let me illustrate this point with a personal experience. Before a spiritual transformation led me to adopt traditional Jewish practices, including obeying prohibitions on eating pork and mixing meat with milk, I loved BLT's, ham sandwiches, and cheeseburgers. As with many assimilated Jews who grew up with "culinary Judaism," food dominated my family's life and I carried on the tradition—right down to the traditional weight gain.

After my religious transformation, I was easily able to give up eating even my former favorite foods. There is nothing wrong with ham itself and I presume it still tastes good. But I had changed as a person. I had a new sense of purpose: I wanted to serve God and do what I came to understand was asked of me. I have never looked back and avoiding these foods never leaves me feeling deprived. Now that's a small miracle and it can happen to you!

People cannot lose weight if they feel deprived. They will find it hard to stay on a diet if it requires forever giving up beloved foods, mother's favorite recipes, and entire food categories such as carbohydrates or fats. They can only lose weight permanently if they feel fulfilled in other ways. If you truly believe that God wants you to eat in a holy way, to be trim, to live healthfully at your ideal weight, it's easy to eat the right amount and not feel any deprivation or loss.

After first adopting kosher dietary restrictions, I still ate excessively. I had no problem avoiding prohibited foods, but my sense of divine purpose did not extend to other aspects of eating, such as how I ate or the quantities consumed. That connection never occurred to me, and my teachers didn't ask me to make it. I had not discovered the Alter Rebbe's wisdom that "what is permitted is not necessary." So I followed the common practice, namely, eating permitted foods to full satisfaction—with the predictable result.

Once I discovered the "secret" of Holy Eating, the power of divine purpose took over and gave me the strength to control not only what I ate, but how I ate as well. If you believe that God wants you to be healthy, fit, and lean for His sake, you can accomplish it. If you believe that only *you* want these things for yourself or even for your loved ones, you may be among the few that find lasting success, but the outcome is less certain.

Human Purpose

A sense of balance is needed. Remember that because we are physical as well as spiritual beings, we remain rooted in daily activities on which our survival depends. We cannot become excessively spiritualized, but must remain grounded in this world. So, in addition to following God's will, identify why you personally want to lose weight. We noted earlier the common reasons cited for losing weight, but let me describe two others that can stimulate you to think outside the box to find yet other human motivations to change how you eat.

A very overweight acquaintance recently lost his mother. His family was in town for the funeral and I looked for him to offer my condolences. I saw a similar-looking but very trim man that I assumed to be his brother. I learned later he was the same man that I had known, only fifty pounds lighter! Several days later I offered him my condolences and explained that I hadn't approached him because I hadn't recognized him. How did he lose the weight? He said he realized that during his mother's terminal illness he had to be fit to take care of her and lift her as needed. Because he had a deep sense of human purpose in his commitment to honoring his beloved mother, he was able to lose a tremendous amount of weight in a brief time.

Sadly, within two years after his mother's passing he had regained most of the weight. What was missing? He had relied exclusively on a human purpose that proved to be transient. His motivation to help his mother was noble, but once she was gone, so was his reason to remain trim. In contrast, divine purpose is everlasting. As long as one remains connected to the divine, motivation endures. That's why Holy Eating yields "eternal" or lasting weight transformation.

My own human-level purpose was less lofty. Like most people, I have always been motivated to maintain health and pursue longevity, despite my weight gain. But over the past decade I had developed a passion for biking, at first biking to work and later making longer rides. Recently, I completed the New York Century bicycle ride, a distance of 100 miles, circling the city in one day (I do only one of these each year).

When I learned that there is a standard ratio of muscle to fat that determines a cyclist's climbing speed, I had a human-level reason to lose weight. More muscle mass, less body weight, more climbing speed—this appealed to me. Those who knew of my passion for biking understandably assumed that the physical exercise itself was reducing my weight. This was clearly not the case, because I had previously reached my maximum weight while biking fifty or more miles a week. My biking habits hadn't changed; my spiritual perspective did. Exercise certainly does make weight loss easier and it's good for your heart, but it is not the vital ingredient of a lifelong weight-management program. Motivation to exercise fluctuates, but God conscious eating can be with you daily.

If you make your human purpose the exclusive one, whether caring for others or personal fitness, you are likely to arrive at a season of life when these conditions change or you simply lose focus. But for the spiritually inclined, serving God remains a constant, the ultimate and enduring purpose throughout life. The sages of the past did not ride bikes or run marathons. They sat for many hours learning and teaching, but they remained trim because they knew how to live with divine purpose—including how to eat.

Exercise

Find a quiet setting where you can contemplate deeply your ultimate purpose in taking on the challenging task of weight transformation. Consider God, yourself and others when exploring your purpose. Try talking to God, asking God to help you define and focus more clearly both your divine and human purposes. Write these below and also on an index card you can carry with you and refer to regularly.

Divine Purpose:

____

____

____

____

____

____

____

____

Human Purpose:

____

____

____

____

____

____

____

____

Spiritual Metabolism

"Man does not live on bread alone,
but by the utterance of God's mouth does man live."
—Deuteronomy 8:3

A common complaint is, "I can't lose weight because my metabolism is slow." It's true that some people have faster metabolism and can eat more food without gaining weight as easily. These people are blessed with this capacity (but will doubtless struggle with some other life task). A good friend with whom I have shared many Sabbath meals always samples each dessert but remains slim because his metabolism is fast. But if your metabolism is slower, this doesn't mean that you can't lose weight. What it means is that you need less food. Don't lament. That can be a good thing, because, as we will see, although eating is necessary to sustain life, it also involves a violent physical process that gradually damages the body. From this perspective, we might say that eating is a necessary evil. "Eat less, live longer" would be a sound motto.

If your metabolism is slow, slow down your eating. Yes, it's easier said than done. Dieters protest that "I already am eating so little that if I eat any less, I will feel deprived and then go crazy overeating to make up for the deprivation." The key is to avoid deprivation feelings by making a transformational shift away from *physical metabolism* to *spiritual metabolism.*

What is spiritual metabolism? Physical metabolism breaks down the substance of animals and plants (the scientific term for this process is "catabolism") and synthesizes them (that's "anabolism") into the complex compounds and tissues needed for life. These processes exert wear and tear on existing body cells, which gradually deteriorate through a process called aging.

A piece of meat is ingested, broken down through digestion or catabolism, and transformed through anabolism into a new substance supporting the living tissues of the person who consumed it. Consider an aging factory in the industrial northeast. The belching chimneys signify that the factory is manufacturing useful products needed for everyday life. But over time, daily production wears out the factory until it can no longer be repaired; it is shut and razed.

So it goes with the human body. Remember the turbulent, bellowing sounds of processing the food after the last time you ate excessively. Many vital organs are devoted to filtering impurities and removing toxic waste. The skin exudes sweat; the lungs filter out carbon dioxide; the liver, gallbladder, and spleen process nutrients and filter the blood; the kidneys excrete fluids and the intestines solid waste. The body has a miraculous waste management system, but the more toxins it must process, the greater the chance of damage. Living creatures passionately desire food because they need it to live. But you don't get something for nothing, and paradoxically the very act of eating to sustain life gradually causes its demise. Excessive eating only hastens this process.

So there are advantages to shifting from physical to spiritual metabolism. Spiritual metabolism involves "digesting" the concepts of Holy Eating into your inner self during the act of eating. The food is not only transformed into new substances for the body but also into new spirit that nourishes the living soul.

The implication of spiritual metabolism is profound. Consider that we eat three times a day and spend time planning meals and buying and preparing the food. By adopting Holy Eating and shifting from physical to spiritual metabolism, we harness a vast energy supply of holiness that can enlarge and uplift our spirit. Holy Eating promotes personal growth on a daily basis with no negative side effects. In the same way that eating carbohydrates or sugar fans addictive desires, Holy Eating fires the passion for God because you are eating to serve Him.

If you cultivate a fiery love for God, this fire has the power to "melt" away your fat. You can create a spiritual metabolism that will put more energy into spirit and less into physicality generally and food specifically. Although you will lose weight, the focus will shift away from food and toward spirit, away from *losing* weight to ***transforming weight***.

The Bible teaches us to not only avoid evil but to seek good. It's a two-part process. Similarly, losing excess fat is good, but not as profound and lasting as the actual transformation of this fat into positive energy that powers growth of the self and the spirit. In effect, Holy Eating does not merely cause weight to be lost, but transforms the fat into spiritual energy, because each act of Holy Eating elevates your spirit. While much will be lost in pounds, even more is "gained." When we lose something, we feel bad and the first response is to recover what was lost. It's more reassuring to focus on the idea that you are not losing but gaining something of value. The goal is not to *lose* weight but to *transform* it into vital energy and longer life in order to accomplish more good in the world.

In my own weight management program, I worked on the most difficult last ten pounds by pledging to donate a certain amount of money for each pound that I shed towards a religious building fund. In this sense, the energy stored in my excess fat was not "lost", but transformed into the bricks and mortar of a socially constructive project. Some psychological programs for weight loss or smoking cessation have used a penalty system that requires donating money to a hated charity if goals are not met. Casting this cognitive strategy in terms of spiritual transformation helps keep a positive focus because the less you eat, the more you contribute to a useful purpose that extends beyond your self-interest.

As the renowned kabbalist Rabbi Nachman of Breslov observed, when eaten in holiness, food can be transformed into prayers and blessings that bring joy and loving kindness to the world."[44]

Exercise

Select a social cause that you feel deeply about supporting. This could be fighting a disease, battling hunger, promoting civil rights or giving to an educational institution. Consider the total number of pounds you want to transform into positive gain for others. Based on how much you can afford to donate to this cause, establish a dollar amount per pound that you will contribute.

Pounds to transform ______ X $_____ dollars per pound = $______

If you know someone in the organization and let them know your plan, you will have a lot of people praying for your success!

God Can Do All These Things

To cultivate spiritual metabolism, you must spend time contemplating the creative and transformative power of God. According to a recent Harris poll, a full ninety percent of Americans express a belief in God. At the same time, as a nation we would get an "F" in religion. In his recent book, *Religious Literacy: What Every American Needs to Know About Religion—But Doesn't*, Stephen Prothero reports that 60% of us can't name five of the Ten Commandments and 50% of high school seniors think that Sodom and Gemorrah were married. This ignorance of fundamentals suggests that few spend time actively connecting with God enough to recognize His full power.

I recall walking to afternoon prayers in Berkeley, California with a Chassidic rabbi who hosted me for lunch. I had delivered a scientific paper at a conference and my academic skepticism at that time led me to express doubts about the religious belief about resurrection of the dead.

> "Do you believe in God?," the rabbi asked me.
> "Of course," I answered, "otherwise I wouldn't be here with you today."
> "Do you believe that God created the universe?" he continued.
> "Yes, I believe this."
> Introducing a more specific theological point, he asked,
> "Do you believe that God created the universe out of nothing."
> (If it were not created out of nothing, God would merely have formed, not created, the universe, thus limiting His power).
> "Yes, this is an important tenet I believe to be true," I responded without hesitation.
> "And do you believe that God created living creatures, including humans?"
> "Certainly I believe this."
> "So if you believe that God can do all these things," the rabbi concluded his argument, "would He not also have the power to reconstruct the previously living?"

Aha! Given the core beliefs that I held to be true, his argument was compelling and strengthened my belief in God's power to transform. Given the many things we thank God for accomplishing—ordering the stars, sustaining life, healing the sick, parting the sea, making the barren fertile, transforming sorrow into joy—it follows beyond a doubt that God has the power to help with a humbler miracle: transforming how you eat. But whether you believe in miracles or not, eating less should not be beyond God's power, if only you truly turn to God for help. If you can forgo eating prohibited foods, never eat meat with milk, or fast for a religious purpose, then surely you can restrain the amounts and types of foods you eat daily.

If you have not yet turned to God for help and haven't adopted other spiritual practices, consider transforming how you eat as an excellent first step. The Kabbalah teaches that a person who returns to God can reach a higher level than one who has been consistently and faithfully connected. This spiritual paradox is explained by the fact that the person who strayed into the darkness of evil actually transforms the energy in that darkness into the positive spiritual energy of light, adding even more light to the world.

A person who naturally has always eaten in a balanced, holy manner does well in doing so. But for such a person, the behavior is easy because it comes naturally. Others can pray or give charity easily and naturally. The person who struggles to eat with restraint must turn more to God for support and strength. Since eating is a recurrent daily event, this person is driven closer to God and is thus elevated to a higher level through the repeated act of eating with spiritual awareness. If each time you eat, your eyes look upward and your thoughts turn towards your higher spiritual power, you add more light to the world.

This reminds me of the rabbi and New York cabby who go to heaven. The rabbi gets a small and modest house while the cabby is lodged in a palace.

The rabbi politely questions God. "With all due respect, why is the cabby rewarded with a palace, while after a life of devoted service I get a mere cottage?"

God replies, "When you spoke of Me, people slept. When the cabby drove, he put the fear of God in them."

Since I briefly drove a taxi in New York as a young man, I can attest to the truth of this message!

The more overweight you are and the harder it has been for you to master your eating, the more effort you will need to put into coming close to God. While more effort sounds like bad news, remember that you will transform more darkness into light. This is something to get excited about: Rising to a higher spiritual level and improving the world—all through how you eat!

Exercise

Every spiritual person has felt God's power operating in their life, sometimes in dramatic and sometimes quiet ways. Write down several events that convinced you of God's power to transform things in your life, no matter how small or large the change was:

____

____

____

____

____

____

____

____

____

____

____

____

Consider this deeply: If God could make these things happen in your life, God can also help you transform your weight.

Don't Live to Eat, Eat to Live

Too many people pass their days trying to figure out how to consume more food and still not gain weight. This is an obvious mistake. The goal should be the opposite: *Try to eat as little as is necessary to live.* Why? Although eating is vital to sustain life, the digestive processes, as we have seen, take a toll on the body that contributes to aging and death.

Eat just what you need to live. This is considerably less than your eyes desire, even less than what you think you need to be satisfied and healthy. Picture filling your gas tank with expensive fuel and topping it off to get in as much as possible. But then, instead of stopping, you keep trying to pour gas in until the tank overflows. As crazy as this sounds, this is what we do when we force more fuel into our bodies than we need to run efficiently.

A study published in the American Journal of Preventive Medicine recounted what happened when researchers gave partygoers either 17- or 34-ounce bowls and had them scoop out their own ice cream. Those using the larger bowls scooped 34 percent more. Apparently, the same number of scoops sufficed in a small bowl but seemed scanty in a larger one. Many similar studies show that the amount we eat depends more on visual cues—what psychologists call stimulus control—than on what our stomach tells us. Our eyes and mind have been brainwashed by food abundance, by advertising that exaggerates our needs, and by restaurants that serve ever-larger portions to keep up with the competition.

As noted earlier, the physician and rabbi Maimonides advised eating 25 percent less than needed for satisfaction. You can achieve this using the cognitive-behavioral tools of *self-monitoring* and *stimulus control.* First, monitor your eating over several days to find your baseline—your typical portion size of meat and carbohydrates that your eyes lead you to believe you need to feel satisfied. Now reduce this amount by about one-quarter. (Don't just remove the brussels sprouts, but also cut back on the meat and grains). At first you may need to serve yourself a normal portion and then remove one-fourth from your plate. Later, you will be able to recalibrate your portion size so that you simply take less. The obvious result: about one-quarter fewer calories with the corresponding weight loss.

Since we prefer to see our plate full and have been trained to finish what is on the plate, whenever possible use a smaller plate. The plate size becomes a stimulus that controls the amount of food we take. By changing the stimulus, we cue a different and more desirable response. This amazingly simple yet effective strategy gets easier with practice. It's a good way to begin Holy Eating because it doesn't require any major change in what you eat and is simpler than weighing food or counting calories. I have found that sometimes even eliminating half of what I used to eat doesn't leave me hungry—or dissatisfied.

Exercise

Consider purchasing a new set of smaller size dishes. This single step can make portion control at every meal an automatic and easy task. Instead of placing the entire platter of food on the table, serve measured portions on these smaller dishes and avoid going for seconds.

Don't Serve Food, Serve God

Remember to transform your meal into a service of God, rather than making it into an idol you are serving. Food is a central part of the ceremonies of most world religions for a reason. It is no exaggeration to view an excess devotion to food that displaces God-awareness as akin to idol worship. In effect, an idol need not be a carved statue but can be a carved turkey, or any activity we value above God. The results of both practices can be hazardous to one's health.

Thoughts are expressed in images and words. To cognitively restructure your approach to food, consider the various meanings of the word "serve." In addition to the meaning of preparing and supplying food, serve can signify doing useful work as a servant, serving in the military or priesthood, to worship somebody or something, or to bind a rope with something to keep it from fraying. But it can also mean spending a period of time in a prison or, with reference to a male animal, copulating with a female.

These various meanings convey a deep significance to the phrase "serve God, not food." When food is served only with the idea of providing for physical needs, service carries the connotations of animal copulation and imprisonment. This is a negative service or worship that is rooted in physical, animalistic needs that imprison the soul. But "serve" can also connote worshipping in the positive sense of serving God by being useful, assisting in a spiritual purpose, supporting God's purposes, serving in a priestly manner and strengthening the rope that connects us to God and life so that it remains strong and doesn't fray.

Exercise

Whenever you serve food to others or yourself, ask yourself: "Am I serving food in the negative and imprisoning sense, or am I serving God?" Repeat to yourself, "Serve God, not food" several times as you are preparing your meal and prior to eating.

Turn Towards God, Not Food

People eat to celebrate happy occasions and so it should be, if in moderation. But a common source of uncontrolled eating is negative moods—fear, sadness, anger, and loneliness. In modern America, when people say they are hungry, they are rarely feeling actual hunger but more often a need to eat to distract themselves from negative emotions. Or they are seeking to fill an inner emptiness from social disconnection and, ultimately, a spiritual void.

When you feel a need to eat, instead of calling the feeling "hunger," remind yourself that you have recently eaten and are experiencing an illusion of hunger, not real hunger itself. Remember that you have ample energy stored in the fat in your body.[45] Instead of turning to food, turn to God to provide comfort, solace, inspiration, and, most importantly, connection.

Kabbalah stresses the importance of establishing *devekus*, which means attachment or literally clinging to God. This might be experienced as a quiet feeling of connection to God, or as a more ecstatic spiritual communion in which one feels profoundly united with God's loving and omnipresent energy. Both states can provide comfort during difficult times, but the deeper the connection, the more powerful the soothing force. Consider a frightened child clinging to a trusted parent; as his or her fear eases, the breath slows and the muscles relax; a blissful sleep may follow as the sense of security grows.

During prayer, pious people cry out to God, "Father, Father, Sweet Father, Holy Father, Holy Master of the World," until He becomes their Father. Rabbi Elimelech instructed his son to call out to God in this way and related an illustrative parable:

> A father and son are traveling. The son insists on stopping to pick some sweet fruit growing in a forest. His father, knowing he cannot stop him, urges him to call out continuously, "Father, Father." He will answer him by saying, "Son, Son." The son, unable to control his desires for the fruit, wanders farther and farther into the trees. But as long as he can hear his father's answer, he will know that he is safe. When he cannot hear, he should run back.

From this parable we learn not only about attachment to God, but also about the dangers of being lured by the sweet fruits of food into the forest of bodily pleasures and of sinking into the forgetfulness of desire. As long as we call out "Father, Holy Father," we remain aware and connected to the higher God-consciousness that returns us to the safety of Holy Eating.

Today we have become increasingly connected to the feminine aspect of God, the Shechinah. Some might find their food desires better quelled by adapting the parable and calling out, "Mother, Dear Mother."

You Are Never Alone

"Better is a dinner of herbs where love is
than a fatted ox and hatred with it."
—Proverbs 15:17

As long as you remain connected to God, you are never alone. But God created us as social creatures that were not intended to live—or eat—without other people. An intriguing theory about the steady weight gain over the past 40 years attributes it to fewer families eating dinner together.[46] Since breaking bread together provides an opportunity for conversation and emotional connection, people eating with others derive satisfaction from what cognitive psychology calls "social support," as well as from the food itself. Eating alone, whether in front of the TV or on the run, is less socially satisfying, so excess eating or other addictive behaviors are more likely to result.

In a classic study, epidemiologists became interested in an Italian-American community in Rosetto, Pennsylvania. These traditional Italians had a typical ethnic diet high in fat but had 50 percent fewer deaths from coronary heart disease. As the epidemiologists studied this community over forty years, although they did no intervention, the rates of heart disease began slowly to increase. The only change during that time was the breakdown in the traditional, close-knit ethnic culture. Children began to move far away rather than live down the street; respect for parents waned; closeness began to generate conflict rather than comfort. The researchers concluded that although diet is important, social support apparently provides a buffer against the potential ill effects of dietary fat. These facts support the main idea of Holy Eating: that it is not so much *what* you eat but *how*.

To improve how you and your family eat, try not to eat alone. Plan family meals as often during the weekdays as possible and begin a tradition of having at least one Sabbath or traditional family meal on weekends. Focus on the connection with the family rather than primarily on the food. Ask about daily activities, accomplishments, things learned, joyful events, or frustrations. Get to know each other better. Positive social support fills the void that cries out in the form of illusory hunger for excess food.

Every meal cannot be with family, and many single people often live apart from social networks. So remember that whenever eating without others, you are not necessarily alone. This holds true at two levels. First, think of solitude not in terms of "being alone," which evokes a sense of loneliness. Instead, think of being "by yourself." Instead of thinking "I ate alone," think "I ate by myself."

A study reported in the International Journal of Eating Disorders found that loneliness resulted in increased eating for people who were dieting. Apparently, feeling alone is a negative state that triggers eating in a misguided attempt to find a sense of connection. But solitude can be a positive time spent with oneself, a time for connecting with you. You are an important person and being by yourself at times can be satisfying. In this sense, you are never alone.

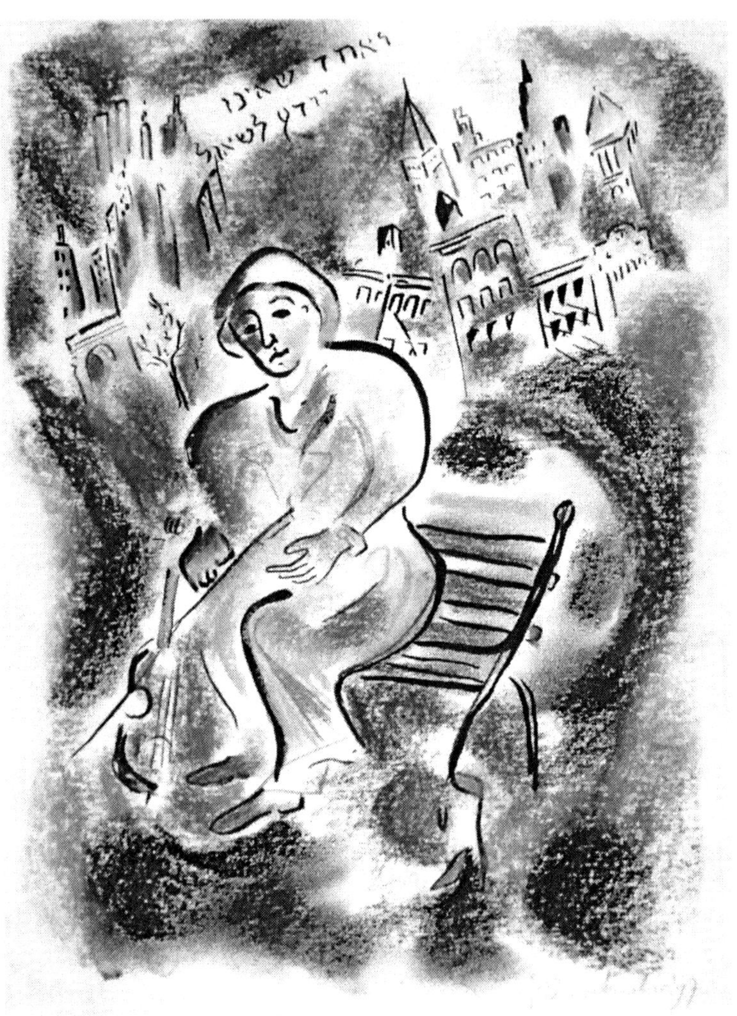

AND ONE WHO DOES NOT KNOW HOW TO ASK

Exercise

Determine if you have trouble eating alone. If so, intentionally set up meals at which you can learn to cultivate being comfortable with the sense of not being alone but rather "by yourself." Use the solitude to quiet your mind and enjoy the good that God has provided you.

Invite God to Your Table

"When the Holy Temple was in existence, the Altar atoned for Israel; today, a person's table atones for him."
—Talmud, Berachot 55

If you bring God into your life and specifically into your meal you will certainly no longer feel alone. Feeling God's presence in your life, in your heart and at your table satisfies deeply, shifting awareness from your physical self and bodily needs towards your transcendent or higher self. Include God in every phase of your eating, beginning with shopping for food, cooking and preparing the meal. Think about the source of the food, about God's goodness in providing abundant resources, and about the radiance of the holy sparks that are embodied within the food.

Many religious traditions promote invoking God's presence at the meal by saying a blessing before and after eating. But even before this, specifically invite God to be present at each meal. At the Autumn holiday of Succos or Tabernacles, traditional Jews eat meals for a week in a Succah, an impermanent, outdoor booth covered with tree branches. They symbolically invite the holy fathers, Abraham, Isaac, and Jacob, to enter the Succah and join them for a festive meal. Why limit this to a specific holiday? Since God is with us daily, we can invite God to every meal in order to provide a sense of spirituality that can strengthen our Holy Eating.

Just as you would beautify any holy ritual, enhance the place of eating as much as is practical for a given meal. Our Sages encouraged us to emulate Queen Esther who made a meal "with such holiness and purity, that holiness rested on each and every dish of food, and on the table and all its utensils."[47]

The table is beautifully set for Sabbath. Looking at the ritual objects such as the silver Kiddush cup used for blessing the wine or the decorative challah (braided egg bread) cover can remind us that we are eating at a holy table. But even for a simple midweek meal, add some small element or gesture to remind you of Holy Eating. Look at a spiritually inspiring picture in the room or place one on the table to keep you aware of the holiness of eating. Before eating, appreciate the visual beauty of the food and express gratitude to God for His kindness. This will make it easier to have spiritual thoughts during the meal and elevate your eating.

I recall during my early return to Judaism watching the radiant glow that surrounded the Sabbath candles and seeing in this aspect of the flame that previously escaped my notice a hint of the transcendent dimension. Aspire to achieve the level described in the words of the prophet Ezekiel: "This is the table that is before the Lord."[48]

Exercise

Remember that since the destruction of the Temple in Jerusalem, the table in the home becomes your personal altar to serve God. Invite God to be present at your meal. Welcome a specific biblical figure that you feel connected with to join you and feel their spiritual presence. Focus visually on some aspect of the table setting and food that brings out the beauty and dignity of the meal befitting your honored guests. When entertaining distinguished guests, you are more likely to eat with holiness.

Washing the Hands and Blessing the Food

Before eating a meal where bread, the essential sustenance, is served, traditional Jews wash their hands and then elevate them upwards toward heaven. The blessing recited instructs us to wash the hands, but the words of the blessing connote "lifting up" the hands. "Blessed are You, Lord our God, King of the universe, who commands us to lift up the hands." While the water is flowing over the hands, we are inspired to think about removing lower self-oriented concerns and appetitive desires during eating. Such rituals are behavioral strategies that help link the spiritual thoughts with actions that through repetition become internalized and habitual.

In washing and lifting the hands we indicate our intentions to adopt a manner of Holy Eating that elevates us into spirituality rather than dragging us downward into crass physicality. We become receptive to ideas of purity, unity with God, God's greatness and God as the Creator of all—including the food that will soon be consumed in an elevated manner. Every material action can be done purely physically or it can be permeated with spiritual intention and energy.

Food is the greatest blessing, so not surprisingly traditional Jews spend much time before and after eating expressing gratitude to God for providing for this vital need. "Blessed are You, Lord our God, who brings forth bread from the earth." Remember that if these blessings are said often, they can become mechanical. When beginning the meal with the appropriate blessing, pause and bring special concentration of God's power and goodness in creating and bringing forth the physically necessary and spiritually nourishing food you are about to eat. In the moment between saying the blessing and the first bite or drink, make sure that you feel a connection with God and a deep sense of gratitude.

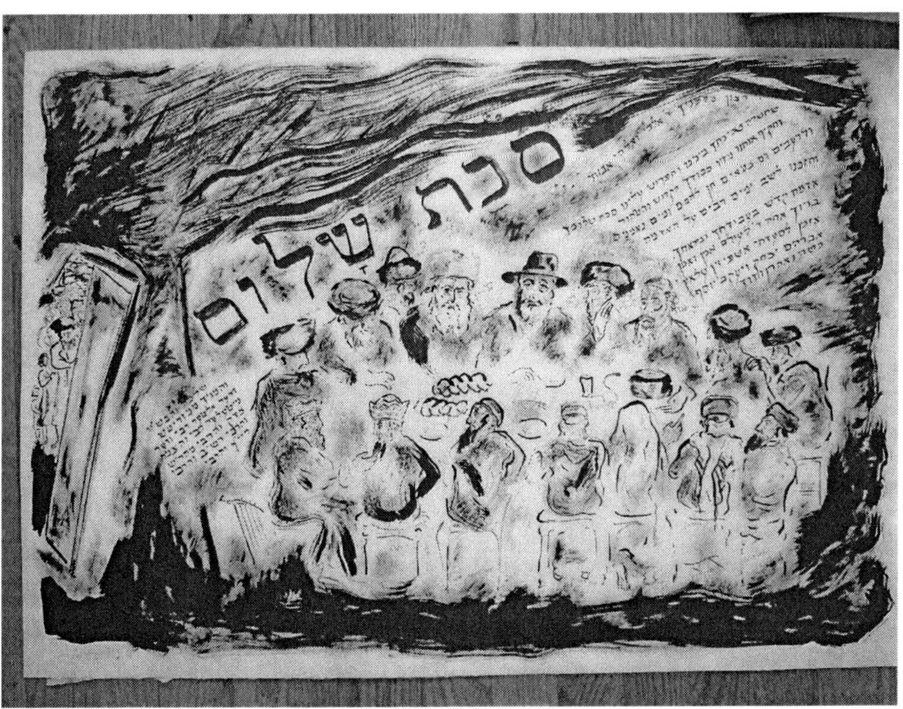

THE SUCCOS OF PEACE (SUKKAT SHALOM)

The Jewish Sages taught that blessings over food should be said with greater concentration and spiritual force than any other blessings: "Say the blessing with both fear and love of God, as much as is possible, especially those blessings over worldly enjoyments. If you do not make the blessings with appropriate consciousness, the food deadens your heart and makes you vulnerable to sin."[49] This is because food and drink have the greatest power to appeal to our coarser natures and lead us to forget God. To counteract this, when you eat try to concentrate on and cleave more closely to God than at any other time during the day.

The great Chassidic commentator, S'fas Emes, taught that food has both a physical and spiritual reality. The more we see the spiritual reality with our mind's eye, the less we will focus on the material aspect with our physical eye. Concentrate deeply on seeing the food with your mind's spiritual eye rather than your physical eye so that your table will be a table before God. See that your desire is also drawn upward towards God as you are eating rather than towards desire for the food alone. In this way, your heart will live and not be deadened, both literally and figuratively.

The Bible instructs us that we will eat, be satisfied and give thanks to God. For this reason, we say lengthy prayers of gratitude to God, the Grace After Meals, after eating a meal that includes bread, the staff of life, and shorter prayers when foods other than bread are eaten:

> "Blessed are You, Lord our God, King of the universe, who, in His goodness, provides sustenance for the entire world with grace, with kindness, and with mercy. He gives food to all flesh, for His kindness is everlasting. Through His great goodness to us continuously we do not lack food, and may we never lack food, for the sake of His great Name. For He, benevolent God, provides nourishment and sustenance for all, does good to all, and prepares food for all His creatures whom He has created, as it is said: 'You open Your hand and satisfy the desire of every living thing.' Blessed are You, Lord, who provides food for all."[50]

This blessing focuses on the God's benevolence in providing abundant sustenance to all so that we can continue to live and praise Him. When God provided manna from heaven, this was to teach that meals should be eaten with calm and obedient faith rather than desperate insecurity about lacking sustenance. Moses instructed the Israelites to gather the amount of manna they needed and not to leave any over until the morning. "But they did not obey Moses and people left over from it until morning and it became infested with worms and it stank."[51] In contrast, since the Sabbath was a day of rest when they weren't permitted to collect food, Moses instructed them to collect a double portion on the preceding day and set aside what they wanted to eat on the Sabbath. This portion was preserved overnight and did not stink or become infested.[52]

Reassure yourself that God provides sufficient food so that you need not eat in fear of deprivation. Negative states such as fear or insecurity, like loneliness, can also increase the amount of food eaten. If we anxiously and chronically grab excess food, we find that we create various forms of "rotten" outcomes such as obesity, increased disease, and shortened life. Washing the hands, saying blessings over food and engaging in Holy Eating helps to balance the body, mind and spirit so these impulses can be better controlled.

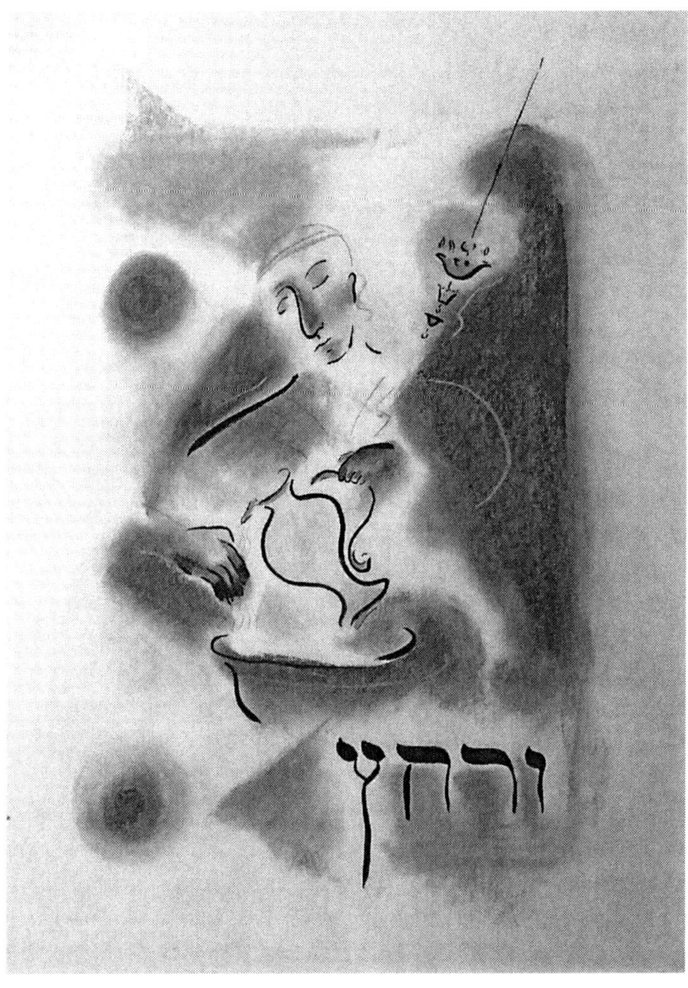

Washing His Hands

Exercise

When washing the hands for a meal, the Baal Shem Tov, the originator of the Chassidic movement, entered a state of deep concentration (devekus) about attaching to God. In this spirit, after the hands are washed and raised, try closing your eyes briefly and take one slow breath so you can deeply feel your hands rising to reach out and connect with God. Visualize your washed and purified hands reaching upwards to receive the satisfaction of your desires directly from God's nurturing love. The purified hands signify your intention to eat the entire meal with holiness. Keep this in mind throughout the meal.

And You Shall Speak of Them

The importance of speaking about spiritual ideas is underscored by the belief that if one eats a meal and doesn't at least mention a holy topic, it is considered as though he worshipped idols. If you discuss spiritual topics at length, you will bring holiness to the meal. But at least make certain that you bring to each meal one holy discussion or thought that is not about material things, acquisitions, business or the food itself.

The French find it déclassé to speak about work during a meal, a concept foreign to most Americans. Spiritually oriented people should not complete a meal without including some holy speech.

Chassidic Kabbalah distinguishes among three essential aspects of human experience: thought, speech and action. Thoughts are important in cognitive therapy and Kabbalah because they lead to speech and action. Ultimately, speech and action are critical because only these produce an actual positive or negative effect on the physical world. Speech is a verbal action that can have as powerful an impact on the world as a physical action. Jewish tradition does not agree with the childhood aphorism that "Sticks and stones will break your bones, but words will never harm you." Evil speech can harm a person's soul and good speech can heal the heart or rouse an army to battle. Thinking compassionately about a poor person's plight is merely a starting point, but only speaking on behalf of the person's need or the act of giving charity will put food on her table.

Because eating is so powerful a force in human life, every aspect of one's being—thought, speech and action— must be aroused in order to achieve Holy Eating. Harnessing the power of thought involves cultivating a proper state of mind, an attitude of attachment to God, concentration, focus, visualization and meditation. Speech involves verbalization to others, self-directed statements spoken aloud, affirmations, stated intentions, and verbal reminders.

One of my favorite sayings to keep in mind during Holy Eating, noted earlier, is the Alter Rebbe's aphorism: "What is forbidden is forbidden, and what is permitted is not necessary." Permission and availability does not equal necessity. We can and must often choose to abstain. Certain foods and food combinations are prohibited totally by biblical law or for one's personal health, but just because a food is permitted doesn't mean that one must partake of it. God put many appealing things in our path as temptations, but the *Tanya*, the Alter Rebbe's classic work, teaches that God takes special pleasure when we successfully resist impulses.

Between pure, non-verbal thought and actual speech is what psychologists have called "inner speech". Cognitive-behavioral psychologists found that internal dialogue or self-talk also can have a powerful effect on controlling behavior and emotion. You can talk back to your excess food desires by reducing negative thinking and repeating positive self-statements such as, "God wants me to be trim," "I will be satisfied with my portion in life and at my meal," and "Please God, give me strength to eat with holiness."

Rabbi Elimelech illustrated the use of inner dialogue as he struggled after each swallow of food between his higher self and his lustful desires. One of the rabbi's disciples was well versed in study and prayer, but he had not yet broken his lust for food. This follower was invited to a meal and was surprised to find only a simple rye bread together with salt (for the blessing) and a knife. After blessing the bread, the rabbi ate a piece and then, overcome with spiritual bitterness, engaged in the following dialogue:

"Lord, Lord, look at how you're eating! Look at the low lust you are filled with as you're chewing the bread, until you want to swallow it in one swallow, and already your eyes are big and you're lusting to chew and swallow the whole loaf at once. Your lust is greater than that of an animal!"

Then he began to reply in defense of himself:

"No! I'm not eating because of food lust, but just to satisfy my hunger. If I don't eat I won't be able afterward to study Torah and serve God, blessed be He. I'm only eating to keep myself alive."[53]

He continued this internal dialogue of conflict after each bite of food was swallowed. This inner battle illustrates many of the techniques described in this book: eating for the sake of heaven, interrupting the meal, meditating about God and eating as a time of battle.

Thoughts are powerful in controlling and directing behavior, but verbal acts in the form of writing or speaking aloud can provide an even stronger and clearer commitment. Stating your intention regarding what you will eat, how you will eat and when you will be finished eating can become helpful fences guiding you towards Holy Eating. Prior to eating, state your intentions to limit the quantity of food to the minimum amount necessary to sustain your health.

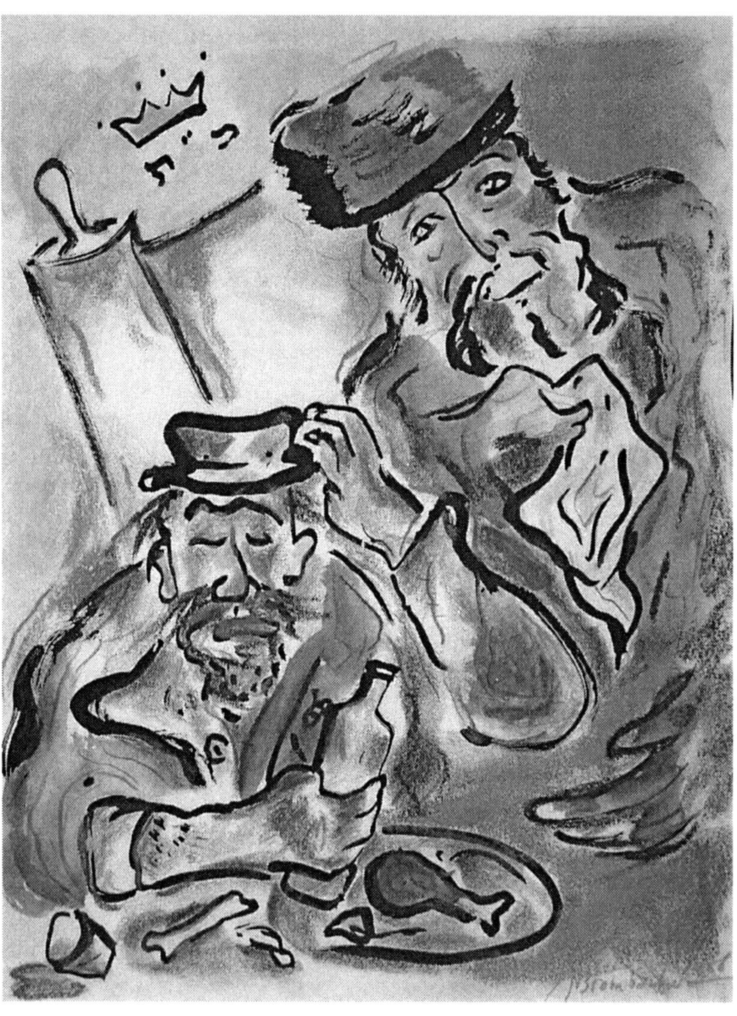

THE SEVEN DAY WONDER

Recall the distinctions noted earlier about the levels of eating: eating like an animal (Level 1 Eating), eating to gain strength to serve God (Level 2 Eating), and making eating itself into a service to God (Level 3 Eating). Prior to eating, consider stating that you will not eat only to indulge your lust (Level 1), but that you intend to engage in Holy Eating to strengthen yourself to better serve God (Level 2). When you have more time, you can state an intention to elevate the eating to a higher level as a holy act. Transform the eating itself into a prayerful act of gratitude to God (Level 3).

When you recognize that you have eaten enough, state you are now finished eating a particular food, a course or with the meal itself. If you are with a family member or friend, you may want to state this intention aloud. It remains your responsibility to adhere to your intention, but a public statement further strengthens determination. One person practicing Holy Eating who has remained trim adopted the habit of announcing, "After eating this next bite I am finished with my meal."

Below are several inner dialogues used by the Kabbalistic sages over the centuries to battle against the animal instincts that undermine self-control:

> "I am eating so that my body will be strong for the service of God."
> "Let all your deeds [including eating] be for the sake of heaven."
> "I am eating so that I can be in the presence of my Father in Heaven, sitting at the table before Him and receiving life from His hand. And my intention is to serve Him now while I eat."
> "I want to eat so that my eating itself will be a service of God by lifting up what is material into the spiritual realm."
> "I want to eat so that my eating itself will be a sacrifice before God, from which rises a sweet scent, and which atones for my sins."
> "May God guard me and save me from my Evil impulse, so that I will not be coarsened by my eating."
> "Master of the World! Help me that my eating is performed with holiness, and that my intention in eating should be for the sake of heaven. Save me from falling into overeating."

Exercise

Memorize one or more of the above sayings of the sages. Before each meal and at times during the meal, meditate on the saying so that it arouses your positive intentions and guides your eating behavior. Develop your own personal statements about how you will eat. Write your original statements and those selected from the sages that you will use at mealtimes:

____

____

____

____

____

____

Interrupt Your Meal

One who eats slowly lives long."
—Talmud, Berachot 54b

Holy activities such as prayer and study should not be interrupted, but worldly activities that can turn one away from God should be. The Chassidic masters advised: "During a meal, when you see that you are starting to indulge your food lust, draw back your hand from it." When eating, one should pause after several swallows, compose oneself and remind oneself of the spiritual purpose of the activity. One disciple of the Baal Shem Tov achieved spiritual perfection this way. He would interrupt conversation to break the hold of "lust talk" or close his eyes to interrupt visual pleasures that were too strong. These cognitive-behavioral strategies involve self-monitoring of negative behaviors and increasing self-control by interrupting the undesired behavioral cycle.

Such "holy interruptions" can break the power of the physical, worldly desires and transform awareness back toward God-consciousness. During eating or other bodily experiences, one can sink into excess sensuality and get lost in the animal appetite. A 13-year old relative of mine had a handsome, distinguished looking reddish-blonde Labrador retriever. He told me his dog was always busy looking for food, but when he eats he just gulps the food down so fast that he doesn't even enjoy it. If this insight came from the mouth of a young teenager, a mature adult should certainly be able to keep it in mind.

This lowest, Level 1 mode of animalistic eating takes one away from holiness. To elevate eating, most societies have instituted the concept of etiquette to cultivate more delicate manners that distinguish civilized human beings from animals. But beyond the etiquette of refined eating, Holy Eating moves to a yet higher level, from civility to spirituality. Try to cultivate the habit of monitoring your mode of eating and occasionally interrupt the meal to contemplate God's generous provision of life sustaining food.

A meal interruption has a primarily spiritual-cognitive focus in changing your mental orientation. But it also has a physical dimension, since it allows more time for digestion. Slow down the pace of eating and chew the food slowly. This will give the body a chance to digest the food and signal to your brain the feeling of satiation, increasing your control and reducing the amount of food needed. Maimonides suggested chewing food thoroughly until it becomes liquid, which he maintains eases digestions and promotes long life. Meal interruption is consistent with his recommendation to avoid eating to satiation, since slowing down buys time to experience the feeling of fullness.

By interrupting food lust, we transform the table into an altar and eating becomes a true sacrifice to God. When you eat with holiness, you may find that you are able to leave a little bit of food uneaten on the plate. Jewish spiritual practices require removing a small portion of the dough before baking bread as a sacrificial reminder that bread, the staff of life, comes from God. Parts of the ancient sacrifices were eaten, but much of it was burned to offer a pleasing fragrance to God. A person who adopted Holy Eating found that leaving a small part of the Sabbath meal uneaten for the first time he could recall gave him a sense of liberation from food, a freedom from lust rather than enslavement to desire.

A Kabbalistic custom for interrupting the meal is to say the 23rd Psalm. If possible, memorize it or have it written on a card in your wallet or purse. This familiar psalm can be applied specifically to eating, as noted in the parentheses below:[54]

> "The Lord is my Shepherd. I shall not want [food or anything]. He makes me lie down in green pastures [fertile land that produces food or provides for animals to graze]. He leads me beside the still waters [He provides me with food and drink]. For You are with me [I am in Your presence]. You prepare a table [satisfaction of my needs] for me in the presence of my enemies [the evil influences of lust, food, negative thoughts]. My cup overflows…[I feel plenitude, satiation, satisfaction of all physical and spiritual desires]."

Sheep are associated with appetite because of their constant grazing. But when the Lord is your shepherd, you shall not want.

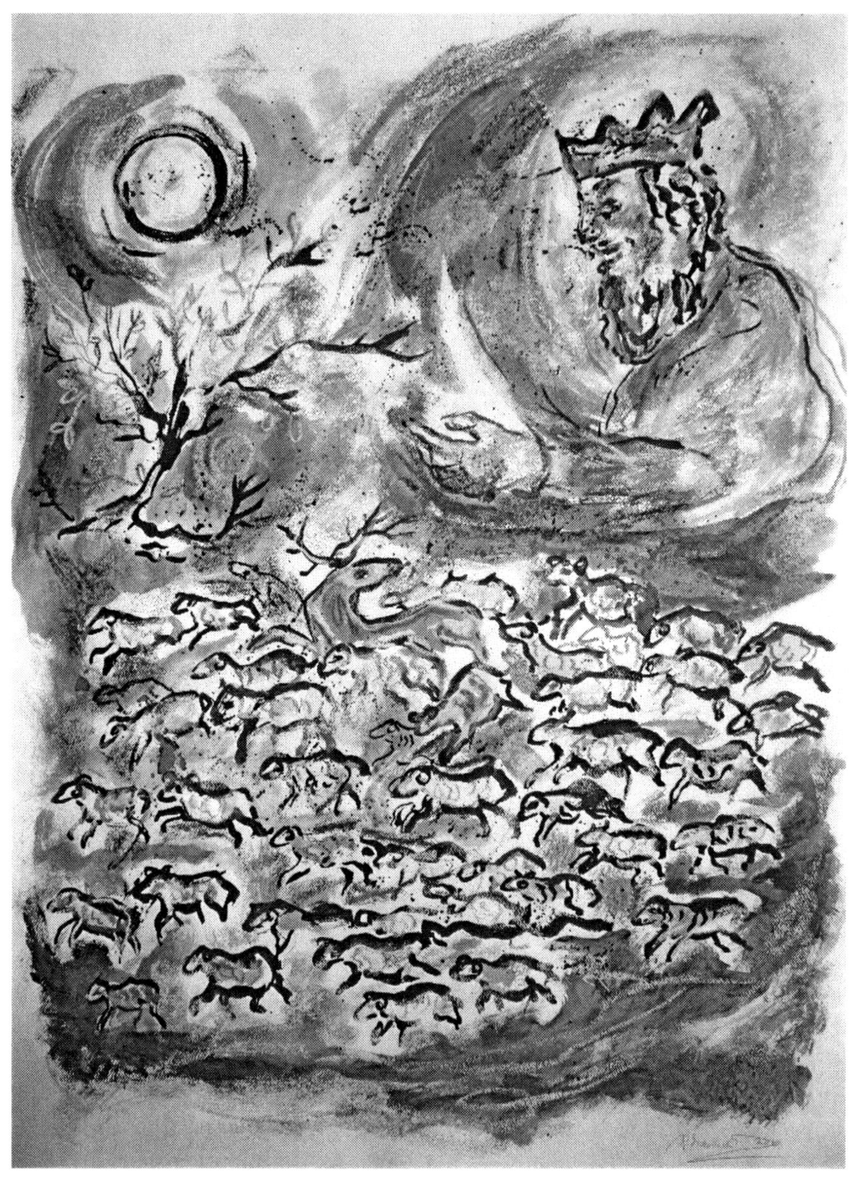

THE STAG AMONG THE SHEEP

Exercise

Periodically during your meal, take a short break. Close your eyes to divert attention away from the food. Let your mind rise upward and bring in thoughts of God. Counter the tendency to sink into food lust and instead remind yourself of Godly purpose of eating. Think about eating in a holy way, rather than eating without awareness, as animals do. Express gratitude or any sentiments you are moved to speak. As you open your eyes, view the food with spiritual appreciation rather than animal desire. Think of the food as vital, life energy, as God's gift to sustain and nourish you.

Transforming Taste

"In the World to Come, there is neither eating nor drinking."
—Talmud, Berachot 17a

Many kabbalistic sages trained themselves to transform the experience of eating so that they did not taste or enjoy the food, at least in the conventional sense. Before you react too negatively to this un-Jewish sounding practice, let's try to understand it more deeply. Sages at the highest level of saintliness do not desire enjoyment from the physical aspects of the world, but only from the spiritual. The physical enjoyment of eating food was transformed by these sages into the spiritual pleasure of uplifting the holiness in the food. What exactly does this mean?

There is a story about the Alter Rebbe who was entertaining a renowned guest. His daughter had assumed the role of cooking for the household as an act of respect for her parents. The rabbi's wife wanted to prepare the meal for this distinguished guest, but the daughter claimed that the kitchen was now her domain so she wanted to have the honor of cooking. The rabbi resolved the issue by suggesting that his wife cook the food and the daughter put in the salt. Since the spices give the food its taste, the daughter could feel as though she had cooked it. Since too many cooks can spoil the broth, the recipe ended up with a double portion of salt!

When the meal was served, the Alter Rebbe and his guest began partaking of the soup, but after consuming several spoonfuls the guest politely declared that unfortunately he couldn't eat it. The rabbi inquired about what the problem was and his guest noted that it was too salty. The Alter Rebbe took another spoonful and completely agreed with his guest, apologizing and explaining the mishap.

Why did the rabbi need to take an additional spoonful rather than noticing from the first taste that it was too salty? He later explained that this was because while in Mezeritch, a center of kabbalistic tradition, he learned the concept of not tasting or enjoying one's food. Only when his guest complained was he then forced to take another spoonful in order to actually taste the food in the physical sense.

This strategy appears to be an extreme contradiction to the typical Jewish tradition of enjoying the pleasures of this world, especially the ethnic emphasis on food as a source of celebration and comfort. For example, Jewish tradition holds that when each person enters Heaven he will be asked: "Why did you fail to partake of all the *permissible* pleasures of the world?"

Indeed, transforming taste is an advanced mystical strategy that veers towards the ascetic end of the spectrum as opposed to the sensualist. Only if one has achieved a sufficient level of spirituality can the physical taste sensations be transformed into spiritual "taste." I do not interpret this to mean that the person derives no pleasure from eating, but rather that it is pleasure of a different sort, perhaps a more refined "cognitive" pleasure rather than a purely sensory one.

For example, consider a musically sophisticated person with mathematical knowledge listening to classical music. Such a person can enjoy the music as an emotional experience and also can appreciate, on another level, the beauty of its musical structure and harmonic relationships. In contrast, a simpler person responds solely on an emotional level, feeling the music more in his body than his mind. The simple listener needs to physically clap his hands and stomp his feet to the music, while the sophisticated listener may appear outwardly more subdued while experiencing an enrapt inner state.

The spiritual person engaged in the highest level of Holy Eating reaches beyond even the cognitive to connect with the Godly sparks in the food and feel the joy of eating from that perspective. If the intellectual and spiritual grasp of the music or food is elevated to the maximum, the experience becomes one of *blissful joy* rather than *sensual pleasure*. The experience still involves physical sensations of sound or taste, but the spiritual subsumes and uplifts the physical to create a transcendent experience.

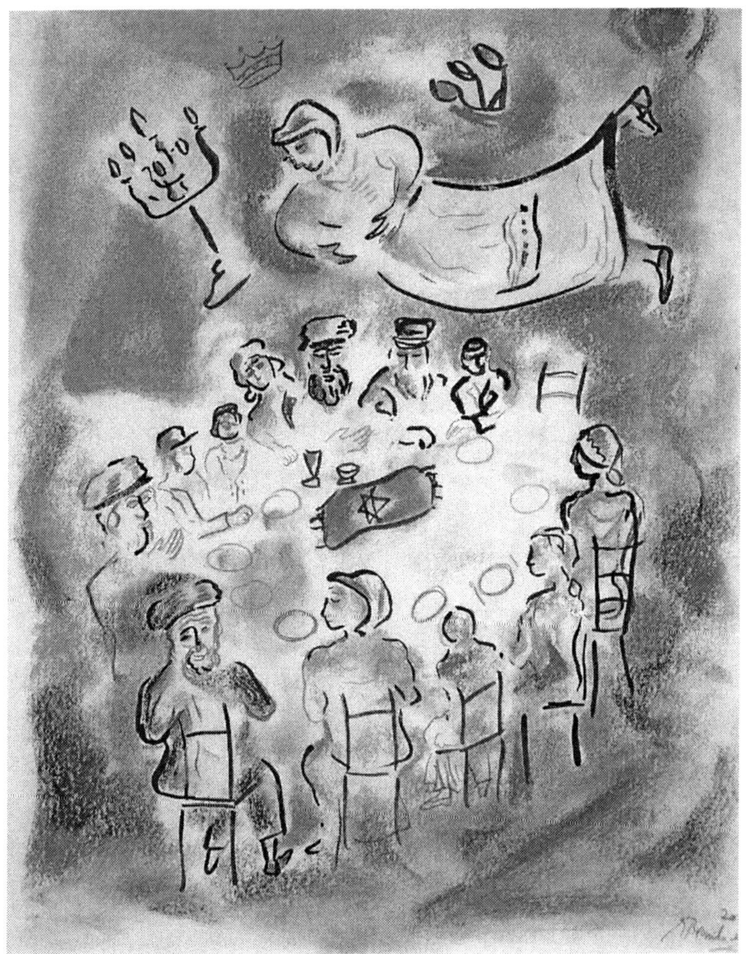

SABBATH MEAL (SHABBAT)

The average person might be better served to partially adopt this practice by attempting to reduce, not eliminate the pleasure and taste of the food. One can reserve a more complete elimination of pleasure for those foods that are harmful to the health. As one develops momentum in Holy Eating and achieves a higher level of spirituality personally, the transformation in pleasure experience can be extended to eating more generally.

Is this possible or realistic? Absolutely. I have almost totally eliminated refined sugar from my diet and have trained my body to prefer my decaffeinated coffee without milk or sugar. Over time the taste experience is transformed such that I now am unable to drink a cup of coffee with sugar, finding it distasteful and overpowering. Similarly, I have so completely convinced myself of the harmful effects of desserts during the weekday meals that they have lost their alluring quality. Often even when I do eat them at the Sabbath meal, I find them disappointing, strange for a former sweet lover. My taste for pleasure is not merely controlled but has been transformed.

As with most mystical concepts, the transformation of taste is difficult to fully describe in words, but can be cultivated gradually through proper concentration and repeated practice.

Exercise

A cognitive strategy used for pain management is to learn greater control of attention so it can be shifted away from the body onto either mental events or external distractions. The less one focuses on the body, the lower the pain. A similar technique can be used to gradually shift your attention from the physical sensations of eating to the spiritual wonders and delights of the food. For example, instead of attending only to the sensuous texture and luscious juiciness of a peach, think also about God's amazing creation with its marvelous variety of foods that provide us with nourishment and delight. Think about the miracle of growth that transformed seed, minerals, sunlight and water into this life sustaining food. As you take the first taste, pause to look upwards to receive God's loving nourishment of your spirit and body. With each bite, continue to focus your attention away from the physical sensations to positive thoughts about God's pleasure when you eat with spiritual connection. You will still taste this peach, but the experience will be elevated beyond sensual delight into ecstatic eating—enjoying its blissful nectar laced with holiness.

Mystical Satiation

"For He has satiated a thirsting soul,
and filled a hungry soul with goodness."
—Psalm 107:9

The ancient Kabbalists pursued another advanced strategy that Professor Joel Hecker termed "mystical satiation" in his scholarly work on eating and mystical meals in medieval Kabbalah. This concept is similar to what I earlier referred to as "spiritual metabolism," a process that transforms physical metabolism by bringing down spiritual energies from above and unifying it with physical reality below.

As Hecker notes, the renowned authority on Jewish mysticism, Gershom Sholem, cited Psalm 34 as capturing the quintessence of the mystical experience:

> "Taste and see that the Lord is good; fortunate is the man who trusts in Him. Fear the Lord, you His holy ones, for those who fear Him suffer no want. Young lions may want and hunger, but those who seek the Lord shall not lack any good thing."[55]

There is a longing of finite individuals to experience the infinite, to bridge the gap between the mortal and the divine. Rather than viewing this metaphorically, Hecker contends that to "taste" that the Lord is good means to literally experience the Divinity on a bodily level. Many biblical passages support this view: "I desire to fulfill Your will, my God; and Your Torah is in my innards" (in my heart or even in my belly).[56] The Torah has been compared to bread, the vital sustenance, and those who eat of the Torah, unlike animals, will be satisfied and not lack any good thing. Ingesting God's law, trusting and fearing Him, creates a bodily transformation of the person that leaves him fully satiated, physically and spiritually. Thus, Moses could survive for 40 days without food or water: "He [Moses] remained there with God for forty days and forty nights—he did not eat bread and he did not drink water—and He wrote on the tablets the words of the covenant the Ten Commandments."[57]

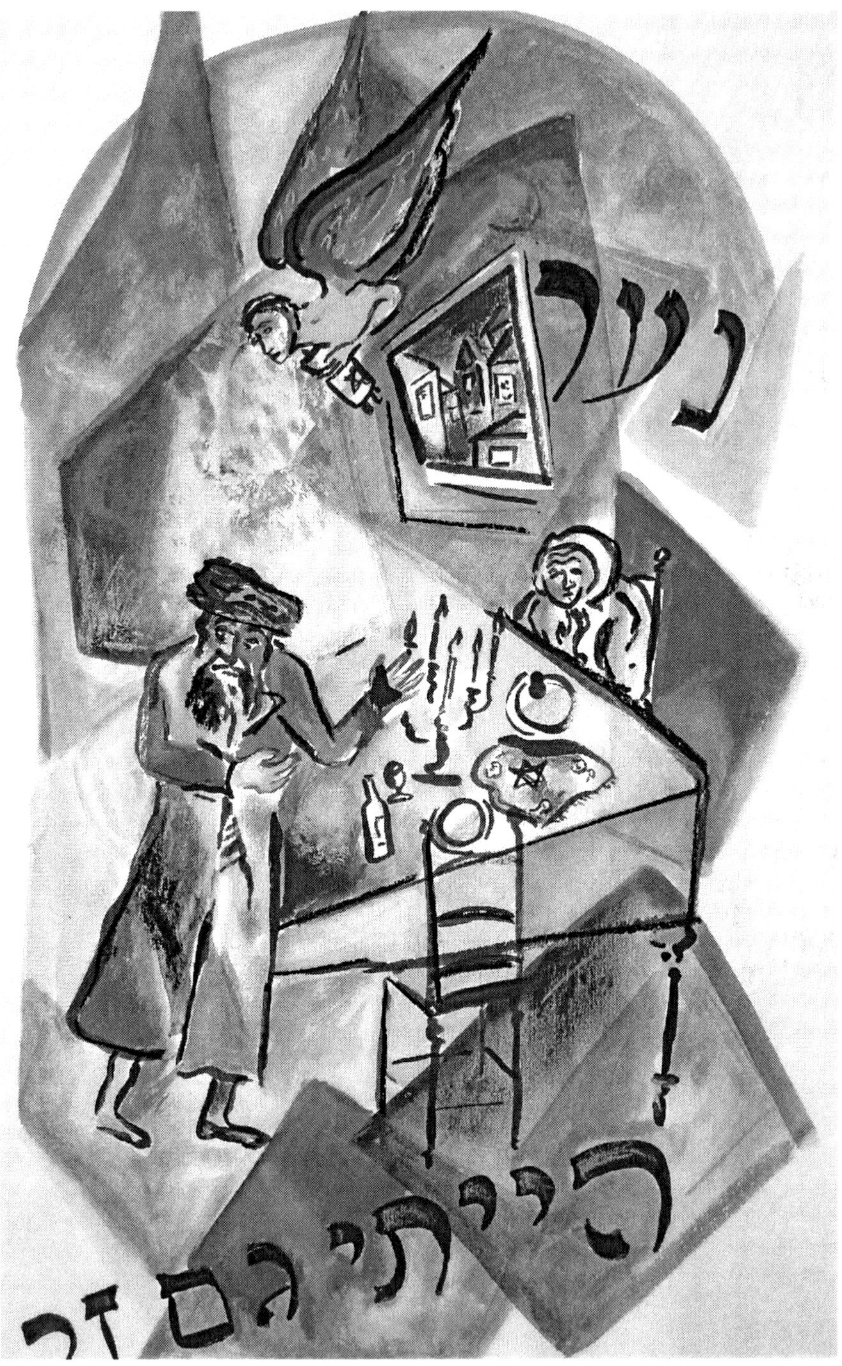

I Was Young and Am Now Old (Na'ar Hayiti)

"I was a boy and I became old, and I did not see that a righteous man was forsaken and his offspring had to beg for bread..." (Psalm 37:25).

For the Kabbalists, prayer, study and following God's law creates a cosmic harmony amongst the universal energies (the sefirot) and draws down these spiritual forces, unifying them with the physical. Eating with holiness induces a flow of these energies to the person's table and creates a "blessing in the belly" or mystical satiation—a feeling of fullness, plentitude, abundance. Kabbalists even believed that one could induce satiation by eating as little food as the size of an olive. This concept is based on the biblical passage, "You will eat and you will be satisfied, and bless the Lord, your God, for the good Land that He gave you."[58] This verse is the source of the extensive grace after meals said whenever bread is eaten at a meal. Since one must say these prayers whenever as little as an olive's worth[59] of bread is eaten, they inferred logically that this minimal amount could result in satiating the person. The Kabbalists felt that with proper contemplation and spiritual concentration, one could induce a feeling of mystical fullness that is spiritually induced but physically sensed in the body. We might say that one can be sated with a morsel of physical food that is seasoned with a large helping of *kavannah*—spiritual intensity and contemplation.

The Israelites were sustained for 40 years in the desert by mystical satiation from eating manna that fell from heaven. Manna, which means "gift," has been described as tasting like wafers made with honey or cakes baked in oil, its taste varying depending on the person's age and desires. Curiously, the quantity of manna consumed by each person remained constant regardless of how much they collected:

> "Gather from it, for every man according to what he eats—an omer [3.6 liters] per person...The children of Israel did so and they gathered, whoever took more and whoever took less. They measured in an omer and whoever took more had nothing extra and whoever took less was not lacking; everyone according to what he eats had they gathered."[60]

The instructions that each should gather "according to what he eats—an omer per person" appears contradictory and cannot make literal sense. An omer was a standard amount of the period, but every person of varying ages would not require or desire the same quantity. But even when they gathered according to what they ate, none had more or less. Apparently, both the taste and the quantity was not a physical property of the manna, but was regulated by spiritual forces that satisfied each person's needs through mystical satiation.

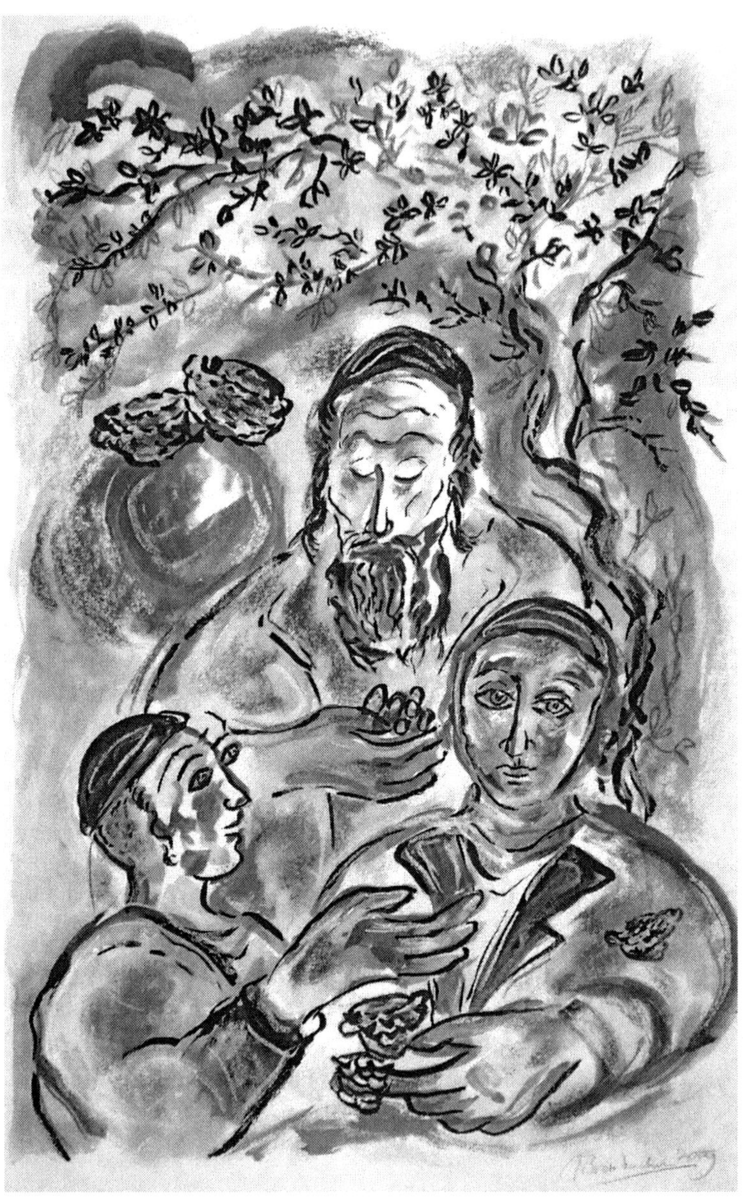

Olives in Clean Baskets, Words in Clean Mouths

Mystical satiation is clearly an advanced state of spiritual practice and not intended as a model for daily eating. But the practices of saintly figures can instruct us regarding a direction towards which we can strive. In this instance, the message is simply that when food is approached with holy intent that focuses on God's presence, one can be satisfied with very little. Without reducing food intake to an olive's worth, try to emulate the model of the Kabbalists within your own capacity. When in harmony with God, one will consume only that which is necessary and will feel satisfaction physically and spiritually. "Taste and see that the Lord is good," and enjoy your "blessing in the belly."

Exercise

You don't have to be a mystic to experience mystical satiation. As you increase your spiritual connection, you will be able to begin cutting back on portion size without feeling deprived because you are feeling more personally fulfilled. Eat a complete and well-balanced breakfast each day. Every other day, select either lunch or dinner (not both) and eat only one-half what you typically eat. Ask God to let you experience a taste of mystical satiation so you will feel content and energized. Leave the table and get involved in an engaging activity, preferably learning a spiritual text. Give the physical food a chance to digest. You will be amazed how easy it becomes with practice.

Putrid Filth

The Alter Rebbe suggested that viewing an object of unhealthy desire as putrid filth can help control gluttony. This extreme strategy is similar to the psychological concept of aversive conditioning or pairing something positive with an unpleasant thought or feeling so that the object of prohibited desire becomes unappealing.

I recall waiting in line for coffee in front of the intentionally placed pastry cabinet at Starbucks. I know that for me eating cakes during the week would be toxic. This is no exaggeration because of the history of diabetes and, alas, slow metabolism in my family. With this thought foremost in mind, I transformed my view of these pastries from delicacies into putrid poison in which I have no interest. I have suggested to clients trying to stop cigarette smoking that they view it as similar to putting one's mouth on the end of a car's exhaust pipe with the engine running. The effect is the same, just somewhat slower.

Yet on the Sabbath when I allow myself a small delicacy to honor the holy day, I can enjoy such pastries. This is similar to the experience of the Israelites in the desert when the manna took on the taste of whatever foods they enjoyed. But some disobeyed God by taking additional food for the following weekday meal instead of gathering only enough for the given day. Because they didn't trust that God would continue to provide, this additional portion became putrid. Yet when instructed to gather a double portion on Friday because gathering food is prohibited on the Sabbath, this second portion remained pure. Eating the wrong foods at the wrong times in the wrong amounts is unholy and results in the putrid filth of gluttony and disease. Eating according to God's will is Holy Eating and provides delight, albeit a spiritualized one.

Exercise

The psychological law of conditioning has demonstrated that pairing two things together repeatedly eventually evokes the same response. After ringing a bell and providing food several times, the bell alone will cause salivation. Similarly, a food paired with a shock will be avoided. Select a food that you currently enjoy, but you know is not healthful such as potato chips or syrupy sweet cake. Next time you plan to indulge, think of all the negative aspects of this food such as its power to harm your health or even kill you. Imagine tasting the food with these ideas in mind and focus on negative reactions to the grease clogging your arteries or the overly intense sweetness throwing your blood sugar into disarray. Visualize the foods connected with repugnant images so they become associated firmly in your mind. Repeat this exercise until you break the lust pleasure for this food.

Submission, Separation and Sweetening

Rabbi Yitzchok Ginzburgh outlined three stages of change in kabbalistic psychology:

> The first is an act of ***submission*** whereby one recognizes that God is the source of all power and surrenders to His omnipotence.
>
> Second is an act of ***separation*** through which one focuses on feeling hunger for God alone and thus distances oneself from all destructive appetites for food, improper pleasures, vanity and other spurious desires.
>
> Third is an act of ***sweetening*** that involves not just disengagement from physical desires, but actually transforming them into a holy purpose or a desire for God and thereby elevating or "sweetening" them.
>
> These processes can be thought of as surrendering to God, detaching from worldly attachments, and transforming physical desires into yearning for God.

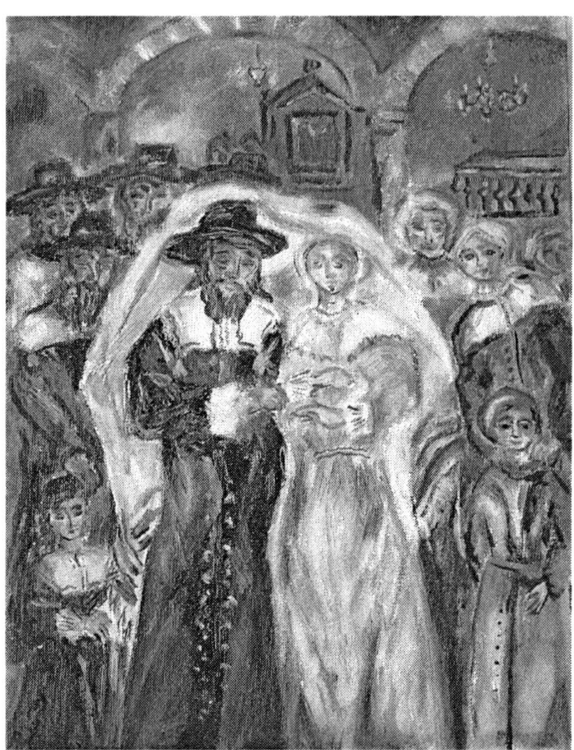

A 17th Century Dutch Wedding Ceremony (Chupah)

Weddings used to be difficult times for me to control eating, especially when kosher desserts that are unavailable locally are brought in from gourmet caterers in New York. The wedding of my close friend's daughter was particularly poignant because he had just received a serious cancer diagnosis. Since I myself had just lost my mother, I was prohibited by Jewish law to attend the actual wedding hall with joyous dancing and singing. I was permitted to station myself at a comfortable chair in a hallway outside the wedding hall.

It turned out that this is precisely where the caterer arranged to display and serve the elaborate dessert table, adorned with sumptuous cakes that were forms of artwork. I generally allow myself to sample more than one dessert per wedding. But the spiritual circumstances surrounding this particular event sparked a different strategy.

I applied these three steps of Kabbalah psychology as follows:

> ***Submission***: I submitted myself to God's omnipotence. I recognized and accepted my personal powerlessness to resist temptation to these alluring sweets. (Those familiar with 12-step approaches to controlling addiction will readily recognize this spiritual step).
>
> ***Separation***: Usually I would admire the cakes in a selective process to decide which ones appealed to my appetite. Instead, I shifted my awareness to these cakes as beautiful creations of God. I found myself focusing more on a detached appreciation of the beauty of the cakes and of God's goodness, rather than the need to consume them. I viewed the scene of others enjoying the cakes with healthy disengagement. Although I was very connected to the wedding event, I remained separated from the dessert table, as though viewing it with detachment from above.
>
> ***Sweetening***: I realized that, as with the cakes, I also was a beautiful creation of God. Since I was trying to shed pounds, by not eating them I was enhancing God's presence in the world, and thereby glorifying God. This small (but not insignificant) act was making my body and the world a better dwelling place for God. My desire for eating the cakes was thus transformed into desire to be connected to God and to do God's will. I "tasted" the *spiritual* sweetness of this scene rather than craving the *physical* sweetness of the cakes.

A Rabbi practicing Holy Eating for several months used this strategy to "sweeten" his experience of the many celebrations he had to attend. He realized that he was not attending the event to eat, but to share in the gratitude to God for the new birth or the marriage. He separated himself from the physical focus and shifted to the holy purpose of the celebration and through this put eating into proper perspective.

Face Your Appetite

"For the hunger is from Him."
—Rabbi Zusya of Hanipol

Rabbi Zusya of Hanipol taught that just as God satisfies your hunger, it is also God who brings you to this hunger and thirst. So there is holy purpose in it. Since everything from God ultimately has goodness in it, we can come to accept a degree of hunger rather than live in total fear and avoidance of it. We learn in the Tanya, the classic work of the Chabad movement: "As the Gemara states: 'The fourth hour of the day is when all men eat, but the sixth hour is the mealtime for scholars,' because they would go hungry for two hours with this intention..."[61] The scholar is spiritually fulfilled by learning the words of God and so can delay eating.

But we can go a step farther. People rush to avoid the slightest pang of what in today's developed countries they erroneously call "hunger" or, even more inappropriately, "starvation." How often we hear the phrase "I'm starving" uttered after just a few hours of not eating. In today's age of food abundance, relatively few people experience chronic hunger. Sadly, a recent report from the U.S. Department of Agriculture does reveal that about 38 million Americans suffered from uncertainty about food and at times actual hunger. But fortunately, the U.S. Food Bank was able to provide food assistance to 25 million of these people. Unless you are amongst this impoverished group, you are not experiencing hunger, let alone starvation. What you feel, however, is not hunger but what used to be called, somewhat quaintly, "appetite."

A cognitive strategy to alter emotional responses involves *re-attribution* or re-labeling physical states in a more benign way. For example, people are able to cope with public speaking if they re-label their physical responses as "optimal arousal" or being "psyched up" rather than anxious. Instead of labeling sensations as "hunger," re-label them as "healthy appetite." We can enjoy a positive sense of hearty appetite, but when we think of it as hunger we want none of it and come to feel anxiety, dread or even panic. H*unger* means a great need for food with the connotation of potentially leading to sickness or death. *Appetite* is defined as a natural desire or craving for food.

This natural desire for food comes from God and is good. Re-labeling or reframing physical sensations is a powerful way to alter the effect of these same sensations. You will have a hard time losing weight if you don't learn to face and even enjoy some sensation of appetite.

The mind is wired to be conservative when it comes to true hunger because this could, of course, lead to starvation and death. Biologists have proposed a "set-point" theory to explain the relative stability in body weight and the difficulty in shedding pounds. The mind strives to maintain a steady state, a set-point, in body weight. Any signs that this is heading below the set-point signals danger and actions to seek food. Harris and Martin, for example, reported in a Journal of Nutrition article that when allowed to eat normally, underfed rats took 6 days to re-establish and maintain their original weight.

Since it takes longer to die from excess eating than from starvation, the monitoring mechanism is asymmetrical and doesn't react adversely when body weight goes above the set-point. This may derive from the feast-or-famine syndrome that is rooted in the hunting phase of existence when prey was difficult to find. When a kill occurred, gorging was necessary because it could take days until the next major successful hunt. Some temporary increase in weight was normal and adaptive because this weight would be lost until the next successful hunt. Now the subsequent meal is at most only hours away, but we still gorge as though it would be days until we eat again.

To gain better control over the impulse to eat, it is not sufficient to only change one's thinking about appetite and hunger. The actual lack of need for food must be experienced as such. In order to establish this new thinking as true, personal knowledge—knowledge that is experientially felt and practically applied—**it is necessary to actually feel the sensations of appetite so we can learn to not fear them but accept them as benign**.

Everything is learned through practice. Young children cannot wait weeks or months for a reward. They learn to delay gratification in small steps, being encouraged gradually to restrain their desires for longer periods of time. During this process, they come to manage emotions of frustration, desire, anxiety and impatience. At first they are overwhelmed by these feelings and either grab the desired object or break down in distress. Those with appetite problems have an inner child that still uses the consumption of food to avoid these negative feelings rather than controlling them mentally. When the capacity to forgo gratification is well cultivated, the adult can manage these emotions and control the behavior.

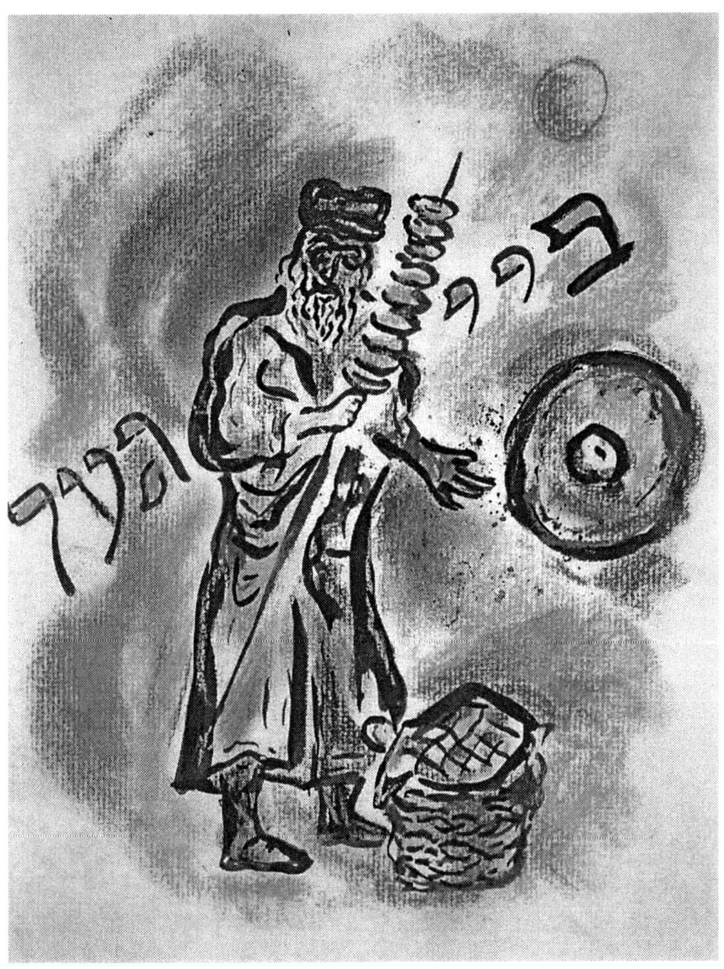

THE BAGEL VENDOR

Exercise

Contemplate the idea that there is nothing to fear in tolerating sensations of appetite. Instead of running away from erroneously perceived hunger, decide to approach what you now call healthy appetite. Focus your awareness on the sensations of your body and learn from them. Be open to your experience and the new sensations you have avoided for so long. Do not fear them. Think of them as friendly and benign, in no way threatening.

What do they feel like, what do they signal? What thoughts do they bring to mind? At first the sensations may cause some discomfort, but gradually as your body and mind adjusts to them, you will become comfortable. Even if you feel some fear, take deep, slow breaths and stay with the feeling until it begins to subside and fade. It will, if you stay with it. Fear diminishes as you realize the danger is imagined, not real. Tell yourself that the feelings are uncomfortable but not dangerous. Breathe and remind yourself this is just appetite, not hunger or starvation. Instead of negative thoughts such as, "I can't stand this, I'm starving," use positive self-talk such as, "I am working up a good, hearty appetite," or "These stomach grumblings are a sign I am transforming some weight."

Now bring God into your awareness and feel His presence surrounding you. Feel a pipeline between you and God and let God's light, energy and life sustaining presence flow from above to below, to your heart, soul—and belly. Just as the rays of the sun on a bright summer day bring warmth to your skin and a relaxed feeling to your mind, let the light of God warm your entire being and bring you contentment and satisfaction. Repeat this exercise until you transform negative hunger into positive appetite. As the French, who are known for their svelte bodies despite a rich, gourmet menu say, "Bon appetite!" Good appetite! Remember that appetite also comes from God and is good.

Contrived Temptation

Once you are able to face your appetite without anxiety in the absence of food, you can next increase the challenge by facing food directly without eating it. This cultivates the capacity for self-control that is vital for Holy Eating, weight loss and just about every worthwhile human achievement. People begin life with the animal desire for instant gratification, to focus on the short-term gain even if it brings long-term pain. Enjoy smoking now, get cancer later; spend now, suffer debt later; eat now, develop diabetes later. Achieving any important goal requires reversing the equation so that restraint is placed first and pleasure is temporarily postponed: Short term pain, long term gain.

Unlike smoking, alcohol use and gambling, eating cannot be totally avoided which makes it necessary to resist temptation when in the presence of foods you may love. The alcoholic can avoid the bar and the gambler can steer clear of the racetrack. But the kitchen or banquet table cannot be avoided indefinitely. So the next step is to maintain control when a chocolate mousse cake is staring you in the face.

Cognitive-behavioral psychology has developed research proven strategies that purposely expose people to situations they fear so they can manage their anxiety by learning new ways of thinking, acting and feeling. After a fearful woman learns anxiety management techniques such as balanced breathing and positive coping thoughts, she is gradually exposed to increasingly larger doses of what is feared. With mastery of each stage of the experience, she recognizes that there is nothing to fear but fear itself. After learning anxiety management skills, those afraid of bridges first stand at some distance from the bridge until the fear is reduced and then progressively go further on the bridge until they are able to comfortably cross it.

Similarly, fear of hunger can be transformed by gradually experiencing longer intervals without eating until you feel the sensations and accept them as non-threatening. Try to relax and breathe into and through the sensations as though you were riding a wave on the ocean. Soon the wave subsides and you reach the shore.

Exercise

Contrive a situation when you can delay approaching the table and partaking of the meal. Obviously, this must be when others are not dining with you at a fixed time. Instead of rushing to shovel in the food, stand back from the table or buffet and visually examine the delectable foods. Notice the sensations and feelings of desire that arise: your mouth may water, you may notice sensations such as licking the lips or swallowing, you may initially feel a little shaky.

Breathe deeply and slowly. Remind yourself of the importance of Holy Eating. Animals rush to the food without awareness, but humans can exert control by bringing God-consciousness to the table. Think of the temptation of Adam and Eve and focus on rectifying rather than repeating their mistake. Focus on the spiritual pleasure of contributing to healing the split between body and spirit, and feel the pride of being on the right path. Let God in to fill the void. Notice that the intensity of your desires gradually diminishes and your emotions settle down. Once you have gained composure, gently step back from the table and begin walking slowly away from the food. Experience the novel awareness that you can say "NO" to unholy eating. Repeat this sequence several times. Each instance of Holy Eating strengthens your mastery and brings you another step farther on the spiritual journey to a more intimate connection with God—and to the body God wants you to dwell in.

Gratitude

Spiritual traditions have long intuited that gratitude—especially gratitude to God—is a key to satisfaction with life. Not surprisingly, research from the newly formed positive psychology movement has recently found that engaging in a daily exercise of expressing gratitude is a helpful practice for overcoming depression and cultivating well-being.

Studies conducted by Rollin McCraty and associates at the Heart Math Institute in Boulder Creek, California found that when people experience a deep sense of gratitude, they achieve serene states of body and mind that can be likened to spiritual bliss. Frustration or anger produces an erratic, spiked brain wave (EEG), but simple relaxation results in a more regular and coherent brain wave. Deeply experiencing gratitude, with both mind and heart, yielded the most profound state of well-being, which the researchers call *entrainment.* In this state, the heart rhythm "pulls" other physical systems such as respiration and brain waves into synchrony. One might say that mind and body are one, a condition of unity that mystics aspire to achieve.

The feeling of hunger for unnecessary food can be viewed as a form of ingratitude. You have what you need but you don't appreciate it, so you crave more. When you feel grateful for what you have, you enter a state of mind-body unity that reduces the hunger triggering emotions of frustration, anger or sadness. So it follows logically from the Heart Math research that deep feelings of gratitude that induce entrainment should also result in less food craving.

Exercise

If you don't have a special, spiritually-oriented meal, try instituting this custom. Make a habit each day of counting your blessings by writing down the best things of the day that made your life richer, more fun, easier or more satisfying. Keep a copy of this list and continue adding new items, both large and small highlights. Share these with family members or friends at your weekly holy meal. You will find that conversation flows, people open up and disclose personal things, and a warm feeling of wellbeing pervades the dinner table. Let the positive goodness enter not just your mind but also your heart. Shift from food focus or discontent to gratitude for all that you have. Mull this truth over, chew on it, digest it slowly and let it sink in deeply.

Chapter 6

◆ ◆ ◆ ◆ ◆ ◆ ◆ ◆ ◆ ◆ ◆ ◆ ◆ ◆

Mealtime Meditations: Talking to God

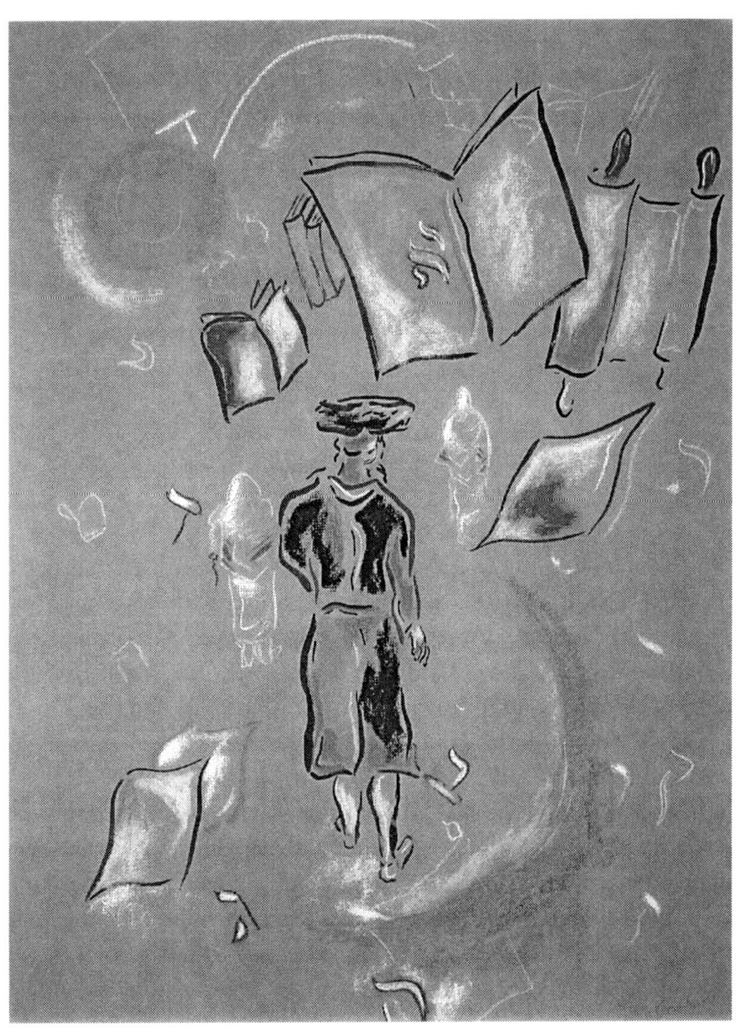

Between Heaven and Earth

Rabbi Aharon Perlov of Karlin[62] grew up relatively wealthy, unlike many Chassidic masters. In order to improve his relationship with God, he led an ascetic and secluded life despite his frail health. The Karliner stressed enthusiasm for Chassidic thought. He was a miracle worker, preacher and a healer, and was known for his vast Talmudic knowledge.

Once a student of the Karliner asked him for an explanation of the verse: "Behold, a ladder set up on the earth, and the top of it reached to Heaven (in the story about Jacob, Genesis 28:12). The Karliner explained it as follows:

"This refers to a Jew. A Jew holds ground and stands firmly on earth, taking care of his livelihood and his main concerns; but his head reaches to heaven, because he busies himself with God and His Torah."

One has to eat both physically and spiritually.

The primary cause of overeating, as we have seen, is the disconnection of eating from its spiritual source. Even some people who have centered their daily activities around God—for example, in deciding *what* they eat—fail to connect the idea of God with *how* they eat. They may have grasped the concepts of "holy" and of "eating," but they haven't fused them into Holy Eating. Or they do so fleetingly and rarely when they need it most—during the act of eating itself.

Even though such people might accept the truth of Holy Eating intellectually, its power to create change will depend on whether they can consistently keep it in mind. Successful achievement of any goal requires sustained focus, which can best be achieved through the discipline of meditation. This chapter provides an introduction to meditation in general. It also offers specific meditations that can be used at mealtime to foster concentration on Holy Eating.

Relaxation training and more recently, mindfulness meditation, have become mainstays of cognitive-behavioral treatments. Most people associate meditation with India or the Far East, but meditation as a means to self-mastery is rooted in ancient Jewish tradition and was widely employed by the Kabbalists. Rabbi Aryeh Kaplan is credited with bringing the kabbalistic practice of meditation to public awareness.[63] The holy sages meditated not only when they prayed but also as they ate. Although they often achieved profound mystical states through advanced meditation, we will use meditation as a form of focused thinking to clear the mind and focus intensely on an important idea.

Meditation strives to cultivate a state of consciousness characterized by full concentration and increased awareness in the absence of "mental static." A person in a meditative state can avoid distractions and concentrate on an idea, word, image, sound, smell, touch or movement. Meditation helps develop *kavanah*, which means concentration or intention, but also connotes feeling and devotion. The term literally derives from the Hebrew root *kaven*, meaning "to aim," so *kavanah* implies devotedly aiming thought and feeling toward a goal.

Once the fundamental idea of Holy Eating has reached a level of intimate knowledge, it must then be riveted deeply into the mind through sustained concentration. Kabbalah calls this process *engraving* because it fixes a thought or image in the mind so that it can be held as long as one desires. A related process, called *hewing*, pares extraneous, distracting images and thoughts from consciousness. Picture a surgeon draping a patient with a white sheet in which an opening exposes only the area to be operated on. The surgeon can engrave in his mind the exact location of the necessary incision while the surrounding sheet "whites out" or hews away any distractions.

Rabbi Kaplan refers to the state of mind that results when engraving and hewing are successful as "locking on." When we are trying to solve a complex problem, it can become the most important thing in the world, and every fiber of our mind and body is focused on pursuing a solution. When we lock on, we can accomplish things that we cannot in ordinary states of mind, which seem to slip and slide through daily activities, making the achievement of goals elusive. Kabbalah calls this less disciplined thinking the "mentality of childhood" and the more directed consciousness learned through meditation the "mentality of adulthood."

Some people already possess strong concentration skills and can lock on to an idea but simply haven't yet taken Holy Eating seriously. Once they "get it," they can implement it easily. If you are such an individual or a skilled meditator, you may want to go directly to the section of this chapter entitled "Mealtime Meditations." Find a quiet place and focus on those passages that most fit your needs for deepening your *kavanah*, your spiritual concentration.

But many who have gained excess weight struggle to maintain a clear and focused state of mind, especially when it comes to eating. If you fall in this category, cultivating a more formal practice of meditation is advisable. You will want to spend some time on the next section that provides a basic introduction to the practice. The initial recommendation is to meditate between 20-30 minutes a day. Even if you cannot do so, consider taking at least several moments before each meal to enter a meditative state of focused thinking about Holy Eating.

You can keep this process in mind by using the acronym *TLL*. It stands for THINK—LINK—LOCK. The first step towards Holy Eating has been to *think* about what God wants of you, not what you want, shifting from self-consciousness to God-consciousness. The next step is to realize and remember the clear *link* between God's will and how you eat. God cares not only about *what* you eat, but also about *how* you eat. Finally, once you have hewed away distracting thoughts and engraved this linkage into your mind and heart, *lock on* to the idea that God wants you to be healthy and trim. Contemplate and use it daily, especially at mealtimes.

How to Meditate

If we think of meditation simply as relaxed and focused concentration, it is a state that everyone has experienced to varying degrees. Natural meditative states can occur while sitting on the beach gazing out at the ocean, watching the waves break rhythmically and repeatedly on the shore, with no particular thoughts occupying the mind. During this *unstructured* meditation, extraneous thoughts about work or dinner plans may float into awareness, but if they are ignored, they can drift out of the mind and out to sea, so to speak. Unstructured meditation produces a tranquil form of deep relaxation that clears away static and inner turmoil, eventually emptying the mind of thoughts and yielding a state of "healthy mindlessness."

A somewhat different approach, structured meditation, brings a more specific content to the mental activity. For example, a person might choose to meditate broadly about a life issue such as a job change, a relationship problem, the meaning of life, connection to God—or reasons to engage in Holy Eating. More narrowly defined meditations may focus on individual words or phrases, visual images, sounds, smells, touch or body movements. For example, the Baal Shem Tov (Besht) retreated into the woods at night to pray and meditate. He became so enraptured that he started dancing and emanated a fiery glow while repeating his mantra Ribbono shel Olam (Master of the World). One can memorize and repeat biblical verses related to personal interests, such as God's greatness, achieving inner peace, maintaining hope during adversity, or improving control of behavior.

I suggest starting with unstructured meditation to relax the body and clear the mind. Unstructured meditation can be done by simply focusing on breathing, counting down slowly and rhythmically from 100, staring at a candle flame or symmetrical form, or visualizing a calming scene. Once the mind is clear and calm, it becomes more receptive to contemplative meditation about new ideas. When you feel more adept at unstructured meditation, you can then bring in the specific, structured meditations suggested later in this chapter.

Preparation: You may prepare for meditation by first engaging in some light physical activity, such as stretching, to reduce stress. After relaxing the body, find a comfortable place to sit or recline slightly. I prefer to sit in a recliner chair, but any position that you find comfortable will work.

Breathing: A simple strategy is to focus on your breathing and begin counting from 1 as you inhale and again as you exhale. Begin breathing in and count 1-2-3-4..., and then gently exhale and count 1-2-3-4.... Depending on your lung capacity, you may find that you reach from 4 to 8 during each inhalation and exhalation. The goal of deep, relaxed breathing is to let the breath enter and exit on its own without forcing it. As you relax your muscles, particularly in your chest and stomach, your diaphragm can expand and contract more fully, bringing in more air with each breath. The breathing gets slower and deeper naturally. A common mistake when people try to engage in deep breathing is to force the air in and out. This is not true deep, diaphragmatic breathing, but hyperventilation—exhaling more carbon dioxide than is natural—and should be avoided.

With each cycle of breath, let any thoughts that enter the mind gently leave. Try not to suppress or actively engage them. Take a passive, detached attitude towards them and let them rise out of your mind as vapor rises off a summer lake on a humid day. As you exhale, let your muscles relax more and more, let your mind become quieter, and let the thoughts and images float away. Gradually you will find that fewer thoughts come, and those that do exit more easily. The mind is naturally active, and emotional agitation tends to generate problems for the mind to solve. The more stressed you are, the more thoughts you will have. Do not expect to achieve a mind totally empty of thoughts, since that is a long-term goal of advanced meditation. After practicing for 20-30 minutes a day for several days, you should begin to experience a quieter mind and body.

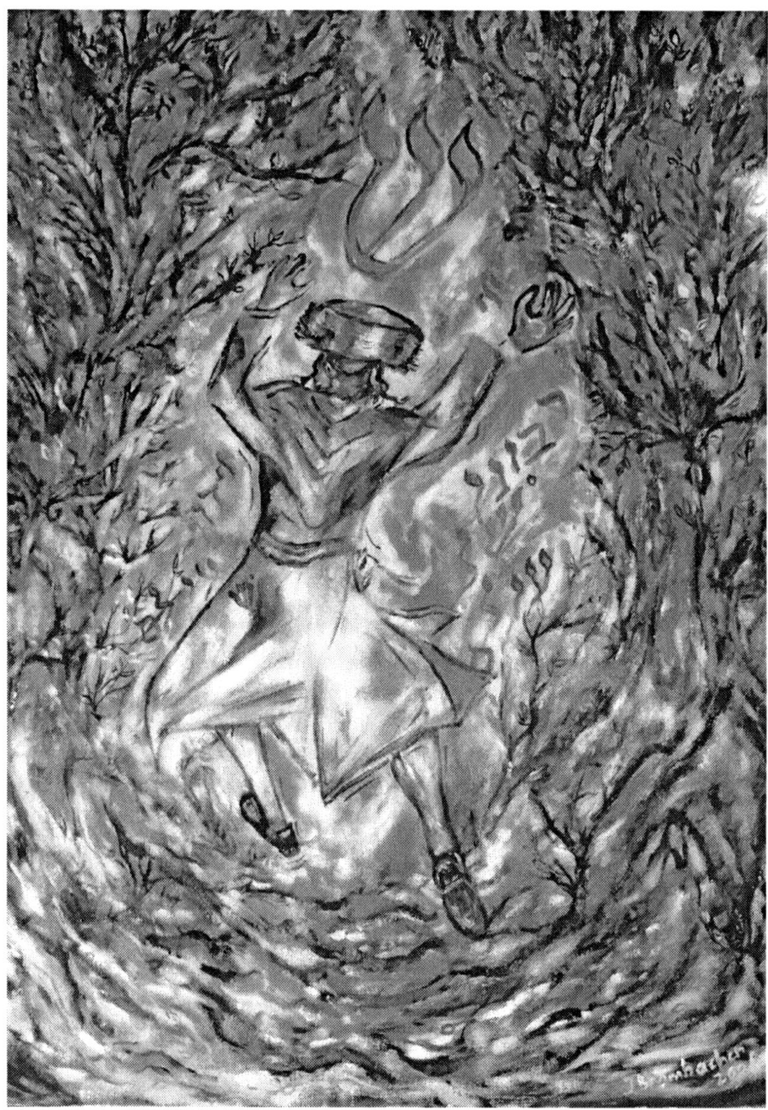

The Baal Shem Tov Dancing in the Woods

I encourage you to be patient because it may take longer than you expect to improve concentration. Those who need meditation the most generally find it the most difficult at first. The goal is to quiet and clear the mind so you can contemplate more deeply and integrate more fully the following meditations about Holy Eating.

Instructions: For each meditation below, I suggest the following steps:

- First read the meditation to get an overview of the ideas.
- Take 10-15 minutes to induce an unstructured meditative state in which your mind is clear of distraction. Like the Kabbalists, gradually hew away extraneous thoughts.
- With this increased concentration, reread the entire meditation slowly and thoughtfully to really take in the message, not just the words.
- Now close your eyes and engage in structured meditation about any themes of the passage that interest you. Let your mind roam freely to discover your own ideas and associations to those themes. Contemplate the meaning that the meditation has for you personally.
- Finally, conclude by repeating key words or phrases from the meditation. Each one has a suggested summary sentence that can be repeated from three to seven times and committed to memory so you can draw on it at meal times. This practice will help you engrave and lock onto the message of Holy Eating.

Remember, a full and detailed reading of the words in the meditations is necessary but not sufficient. It is important to weave the emotional impact of the words into your own subjective experience, your deeper self, so it becomes intimate and passionate wisdom.

Mealtime Meditations

Focus on God

God created the universe and is re-creating it at every moment. God constantly directs His energy toward sustaining the world. This is especially evident in the amazing cycle of food production that draws on God's gifts of light, water, and earth. Without God's concentration for even a moment, the world would cease to exist. Since meditation is a form of intense concentration or focus, we might say that God meditates on His creations constantly.

Emulate God. Focus your attention on God and keep Him in constant awareness, as He does for you. We can express our gratitude to God by maintaining awareness of the way in which He brings the universe into being and generally supplies food in abundance. As noted earlier, focused awareness of God is most important when eating because this physical act can so easily distract us from spirituality. Whenever you eat, more than at any other time, concentrate your mind deeply on God and let your heart cleave more closely to Him. Feel God's presence in all His works; let everything you see, hear, feel, smell, and touch remind you of Him. Especially when you are eating, an act that stimulates all your senses, see God's Hand in every stage of creating, preparing, consuming, and even eliminating the food. Be aware and remind yourself. Concentrate.

Meditation:
I will keep God before me always.
I think of You continually and especially when eating.
As the poet saw infinity in a grain of sand,
I see Your divine love in my daily bread.
I invite you to my table at every meal.
I will eat only to serve You better,
and elevate the sparks in the food
through Holy Eating.
As You are holy, I will eat with holiness.

Repeat: I see Your divine love in my daily bread.

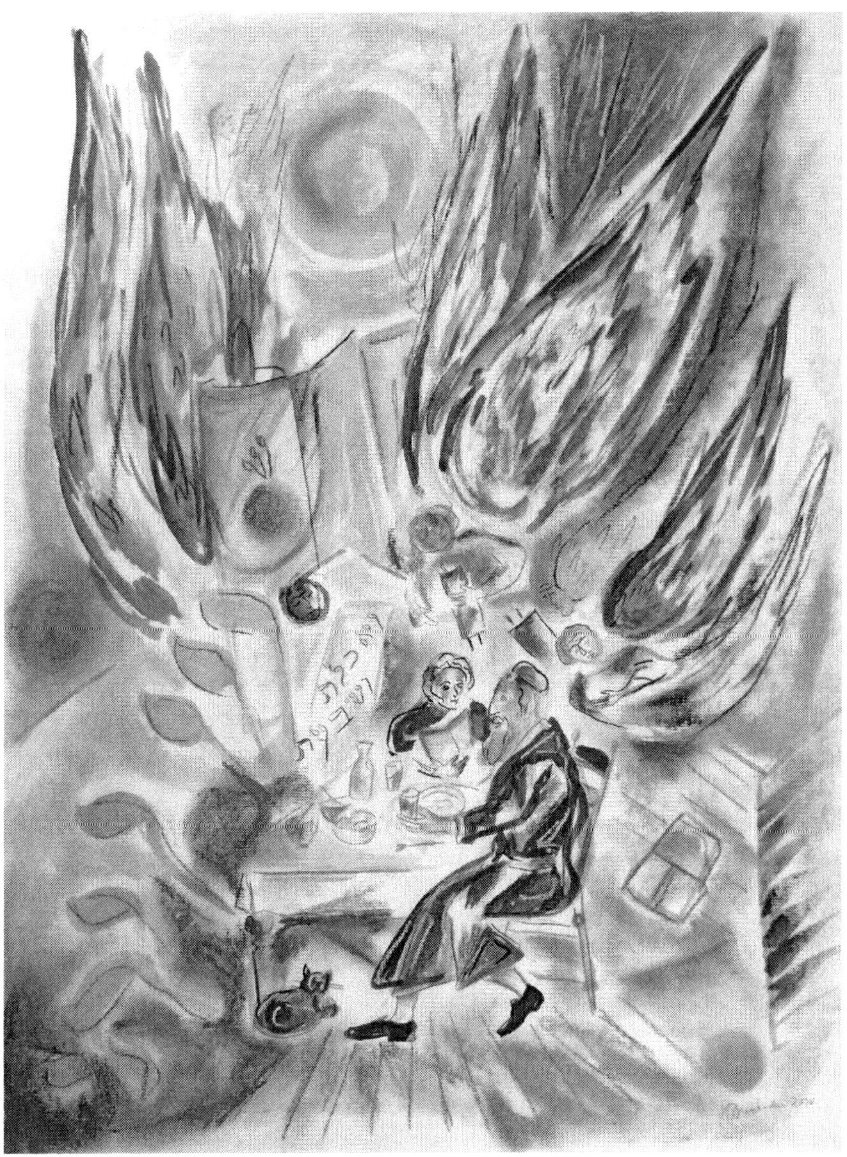

Shiviti (Set Before Me)

"I have set (shiviti) the Lord always before me."
—(Psalm 16:8)

God Loves You

The essential idea of Holy Eating is that because God cares about his creations, He wants them to experience His goodness and to be healthy. The Kabbalah teaches that the spiritual energies, or *sefirot,* that emanate from God flow first through the intellectual faculties and next through the emotions. The primary emotions are love, kindness, and overflowing expansiveness. The Kabbalists stated that God created the universe in order to express love, and the renowned Rabbi Akiva affirmed that this love is a cardinal principle in the Bible. But since love is reciprocal, we must also feel and express this love toward God. The central Jewish prayer, the *Shemah*, reminds us of this sacred obligation: "You shall love the Lord your God with all your heart, with all your soul, and with all your might."

The primary motivation for losing weight is not that *you* want to be healthy, but rather that *God* loves you and wants you to be healthy. You can feel this love by strengthening your connection with God through meditating on God's greatness and by following His will.

Love comes in two forms: *unconditional* and *conditional*. God loves you unconditionally, regardless of how you act or look, but at another level He wants you to walk in His ways, to act according to His will. Good parents expect certain behaviors from their children, but they still love them unconditionally when they stray. Remember that God loves you as you are unconditionally, even though at the same time He wants you to improve yourself continually. You are never totally cut off from God's love, but you can always connect more closely. The more we feel connected to God, the more spiritual fulfillment we derive. This is the first and foremost idea to engrave into the mind.

Rabbi Aryeh Kaplan illustrated the power of God's love by comparing it to that felt by human lovers. Recall when you and your beloved first met. You yearned to be together and thought of each other often when apart. The goal of lifelong partners in love is to sustain this state of enthusiasm. Focusing on the love of God can keep God-consciousness steadfastly in mind. This awareness comes to pervade all our activities, from the most spiritual, such as praying and giving charity, to the physical, such as dressing, walking, and, of course, eating. As Maimonides advised, we should love God as "One who is love-sick and cannot take his mind off the woman he loves, but always thinks of her when lying down or rising up, when eating or drinking" (cited in Buxbaum, p. 267).

Meditation:
God of love,
inspire my mind, comfort my soul, and satisfy my body.
I strive to draw closer to You
and yearn to connect with Your Divine presence.
Dear God, embrace me with Your love
and envelop me in Your light.
Your love sustains and satisfies me.
When I feel Your love, I know no hunger.
My cup is truly full.
From Your love flows warmth, goodness, sustenance,
security, abundance, and joy.
Renew my enthusiasm for You constantly,
so I shall remain steadfast in my love for You
and unswerving in my devotion to do Your will.

Repeat: My cup is full and I am satisfied through Your love and Your light.

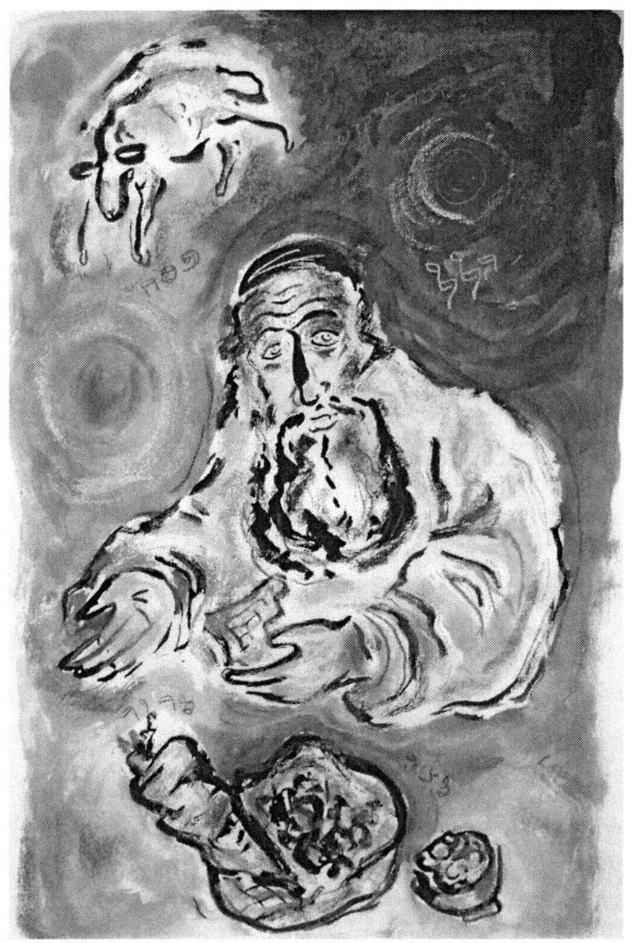

THE HILLEL SANDWICH

During the Passover seder matzah is eaten together with maror (bitter herbs) and the symbols of Passover are mentioned. This is called the Hillel sandwich, after Rabbi Hillel (110 BCE to 10 CE) who was associated with the development of the Talmud and famously said, "If I am not for myself, who will be for me? If I am only for myself, what am I? And if not now, when?"

Awe of God

Kabbalah teaches that the universal spiritual energies comprise polar opposites that must be harmonized or brought into balance. The energy associated with justice, separation, and restriction, stands in opposition to loving-kindness. Love cannot expand endlessly without boundaries but must be balanced by restraint. On the other hand, an extreme state of restriction, justice without mercy, would destroy the world. Who could withstand undiluted judgment and survive? An energy called harmony or beauty is the unifying force that strikes a balance between all apparent contradictions, including undiluted love and merciless justice. The path of God is the middle path between these opposing dualities.

We can only approach God's love up to a point. We must also stand back with a respectful distance, in reverential awe. God wants to bestow His love upon us, but He also must chastise us, and awe reminds us of this reality. Awe, often misunderstood as fear, is not a purely negative state. Rather, awe of God is a more complex emotion that includes fear, but also amazement, respect, and reverence, mixed with feelings of personal insignificance and powerlessness.

The emphasis of Holy Eating is on feeling a connection through God's love, but this love must be balanced with awe that underscores a respectful distance. Although ordinary subjects might dine with a King or Queen, they must remain appropriately respectful. Meditating on the greatness and overflowing goodness of God arouses within us not only a love of God but also a profound sense of awe. The love reminds us of the nourishing and life-preserving value of Holy Eating. The awe reminds us to set limits on the type and amount of food we eat, cautioning us to include only what is healthy and to exclude that which harms.

This truth can be seen most clearly in relation to eating, where too much of a good thing can be deadly. God can provide abundant food, but if we do not accept limits and overindulge in this goodness, this very same food can poison and destroy us. When the Israelites collected more manna than instructed or yearned for meat rather than enjoying what God provided, God's wrath struck them down because of their gluttony. I cite this biblical precedent not to induce excess guilt or fear, which are counterproductive to maintaining control, but only to acknowledge the reality that God motivates through both love and awe. Humans need both the carrot and the stick. Similarly, when the awe of God makes us feel powerless, we should not dwell on feeling impotent and lost, but rather on feeling encouraged to turn reverentially toward God and to more fully connect with His amazing power. It is this power, more than our own, that will win the battle against overeating.

Meditation
I know that you love all your creations,
but at times I fear Your awesome power
and stand trembling before You.
You create darkness as well as light,
and bring forth both death and life.
Forgive my unholy eating
that distances me from You.
God of justice,
free me from the snare of gluttony,
give me the wisdom to choose life,
and the strength to follow
Your holy path.

Repeat: God of awe and justice, give me the wisdom to choose life and the strength to follow Your holy path.

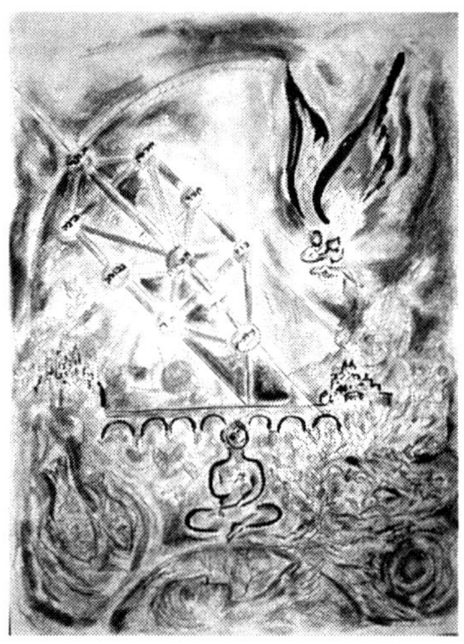

THE SEFIROT

A man is meditating upon the kabbalistic tree of the ten Sefirot, the spiritual principles which form the Universe, surrounded by the symbols of the four basic elements: earth, water, air, fire.

How Satiating is Your Kindness

"Taste and see that the Lord is good."
—Psalm 34:9

"Not by bread alone does a man live
but by every word that proceeds
out of the mouth of the Lord"
—Deuteronomy 8:3

As noted earlier, the medieval Kabbalists cultivated a state of mystical satiation. This allowed them to feel a "blessing in the belly" through spiritual connection that satisfied physical hunger with minimal amounts of actual food. Holy Eating strives to fire up "spiritual metabolism" such that the more connected you feel to God, the less craving you have for anything else, including food.

You may meditate on any spiritual passage (such as Psalm 23) that fosters a deep bond with God. I experience this connection on a regular basis from saying several verses from Psalm 36 (8:1) when I drape myself in the prayer shawl in preparation for morning prayers:

"How precious is your kindness, O God! The children of men take refuge in the shadow of Your wings. They shall be *satiated with the delight of Your House*, and You will give them to *drink from the river of Your bliss.* For with you is the source of life; in your light we will see light. Bestow Your kindness upon those who know you, and Your righteousness on the upright in heart [italics added]."

Meditation:
Let me be sheltered in the shadow of God's wings,
safe and secure.
Open my heart to the true source of satisfaction and nourishment.
God, in Your expansiveness
provide me with abundance, delight, joy and bliss.
Open my heart to feel this flow of abundance
and to be satiated with loving kindness.
In Your light, I see the source of life.
By absorbing the light, I draw an endless flow of energy, vitality, and strength.

Although the sun is millions of miles away, its rays travel to meet me personally.
God is both distant and close,
Off in supernal realms, yet touching me through this light.
I feel the warm radiance and
absorb it deeply into my body, self and soul.
Dear God, let the Divine light enter my belly and be a blessing of contentment and satisfaction.
Let there be abundant light within me.

Repeat: Source of life and light: Shelter me in the shadow of Your wings, satiate me with Your delights and let me drink from the river of Your bliss.

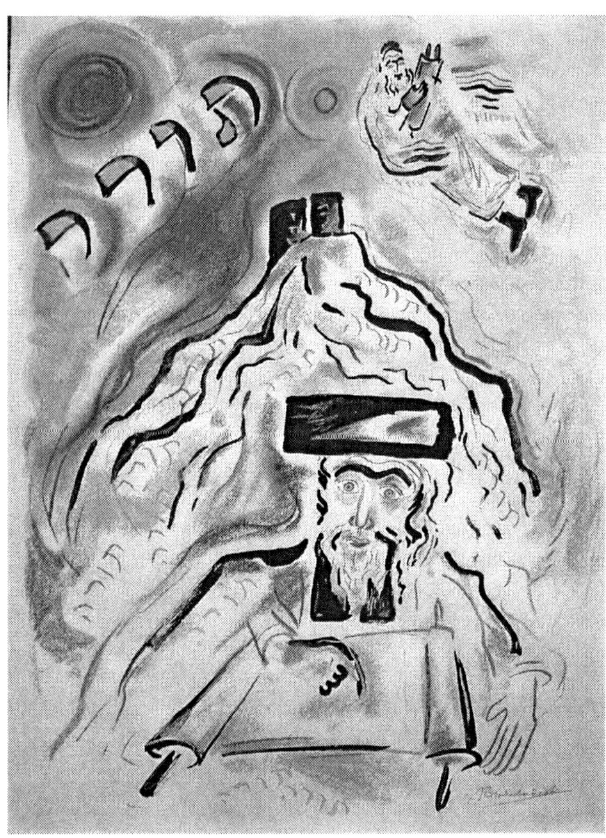

TORAH

Food at the Proper Time

"The eyes of all look expectantly to You, and You give them their food at the proper time. You open Your hand and satisfy the desire of every living thing. The Lord is righteous in all His ways, and benevolent in all His deeds. The Lord is close to all who call upon Him, to all who call upon Him in truth."
—Psalm 145: 15-18

God gives you food at the *proper* time, not merely when you desire it or when you think it is proper. God knows the amount and time that is appropriate. Just as God counts the stars in the heaven and orders every detail of the universe to maintain balance and harmony, so He provides the right amount of food at the right time for you. Consider this when you eat and open your mind to the truth about what *you* think you need and what *God* knows is your proper portion. Humbly ask God to guide you to find this proper manner of eating.

Meditation:
Dear God, I know that my eyes often covet
more food than my stomach needs.
Please open my eyes
and remove this falsehood,
so I can see Your will more clearly.
Give me food at the proper time
and let my portions be balanced.
Open Your Hand, dear God,
satisfy my desires,
and guide me to eat with holiness.

Repeat: Open my eyes to see that You give me food at the proper time and in the proper amount. Open Your hand and satisfy all my desires.

God Is Everywhere

I asked someone who had been trying to lose weight how it was going. "It *was* going well, but then I went on vacation to California and lost focus," she replied. "I haven't been able to get back on track since I returned. Problems at work and the usual hassles with my husband have stressed me out."

This is the universal experience of people trying to lose weight: Something always comes up in life, either positive events like a vacation cruise, a wedding, or holiday meals, or negative ones like work stress, personal conflict, or financial worry. These draw attention from the diet, and what was to be a temporary lapse becomes a complete relapse.

The beauty of Holy Eating is that God is everywhere. This includes your exotic vacation destination and even that remote stretch of unpopulated wilderness through which you may travel. God is with you on the cruise. God is at your holiday meal. God is especially with you during your stressful times of sorrow, loss, and pain. Without the continuous awareness of the presence of God, it is nearly impossible for most people to maintain a continuous process of successful weight management.

People want to celebrate positive events with food and comfort themselves during hard times with food. We create the illusion that these times are exceptions so we can sneak in some indulgence without doing harm. Everyone has heard the line about desserts not having calories at Sabbath meals. But they do, because God and His laws are operating also at that time. Physical metabolism is the same in all times and places, but you can shift to spiritual metabolism when you remember that God is everywhere. This applies to every meal, at every table, in every location in the universe, and for every bite.

Understand that God is everywhere, in everything.

Look for Him for He is concealed in everything you do and can be revealed at every moment.

Maintain practices that keep God in your awareness at all times.

Look towards Heaven in whatever you do, and you will be prepared for all of life's difficult moments of choice, including eating.

Meditation:
Wherever I am, Lord,
You are with me.
Your presence permeates my home
and Your spirit secures my journey.
You are with me in sorrow and celebration.
I will not hide from You, nor sneak in vain,
but strive to stay constantly connected
to Your satiating light.
Through Holy Eating,
I will seek You everywhere
and remember You with every bite.

Repeat: Wherever I go, I seek Your satiating light and remember You with every bite.

I Am Weak, Strengthen Me

"He gives food to the hungry;
the Lord releases those who are bound."
—Psalm 146:7

Some of us have felt moved to make pleas such as the these:

"Oh, God, I am bound, imprisoned by my false hunger and unfulfilled desires. I come to you trembling with hunger and weakness, out of control of my eating. I have been enslaved by food, rather than serving You. My weight bears down heavily upon me."

"I yearn for connection, but it escapes me. I crave love, but it doesn't reach me. Dear God, soften my heart so that I can let You in. May I feel Your comforting love and warm presence. Release me from my bondage and satisfy my hunger."

"Please, God, return me to Your path of balance, moderation, and health. Instill within me Your power and strength. When I connect with You, I feel steady and strong, clear in mind, and ready to serve You, rather than enslaved by food. The food you provide for me gives me renewed strength, energy, and vigor. As I chew and swallow, I enjoy the pleasurable taste and the enlivening effect on my body. I know that You provide this sustenance because of Your love for me, as a parent loves and nourishes a son or daughter. "

The following meditation addresses such concerns:

Meditation:
I indulged gluttonously,
but you teach me the path of moderation.
Please transform my food lust
into holy passion,
my excess weight
into positive energy.
Thank you, God, for helping me
control my desire for food.

I am bound,
but You will set me free.
I am weak,
but you give me strength.
I know that You desire health for all your creations
and Holy Eating will render me whole.

You give me courage and might.
Thank you, God, for uniting my will with Yours.

Repeat: Dear God, transform my weakness into strength, my food lust into holy passion, my excess weight into positive energy. Unite my will with Your will.

Let Food Elevate You, Not Weigh You Down

When we eat lustfully, without God-consciousness, the soul sinks down into a physical, animal state. But when we eat with awareness that the food is from God, the food becomes a ladder to higher spiritual joy and connection with God. If ordinarily you derive so much pleasure from the physical aspects of food, think of the unlimited pleasure when you taste the "holy sparks" that come from the ultimate Source and Creator of the food. A wise person who is sitting in the dark and sees a small beam of light shining under a closed door will not be content with only this beam. Instead he will open the door to find the source of light.

Before eating, close your eyes for a few moments and meditate on God's power to elevate and to bring forth food. Be aware that God is constantly present, so you will eat with the dignity that befits this holy guest. When you bite into the luscious fruit or favorite meal, derive your pleasure. However, let this pleasure be not only sensual, but also infused with spiritual awareness, with God-consciousness.

Meditation:
Dear God, I invite You to my table.
I will look beyond the surface of the food,
and seek within it the holy sparks
of Your presence.
Let eating elevate my spirit
and not weigh down my body.
I will enjoy the pleasure of food,
but I remind myself that the greatest pleasure
is my attachment to You.
Let the sensual pleasure of food
be permeated with the spiritual pleasure
of knowing that all I eat comes from Your Hand.
Let my eating be with holiness.

Repeat: I will elevate my eating and constantly seek the holy sparks in food.

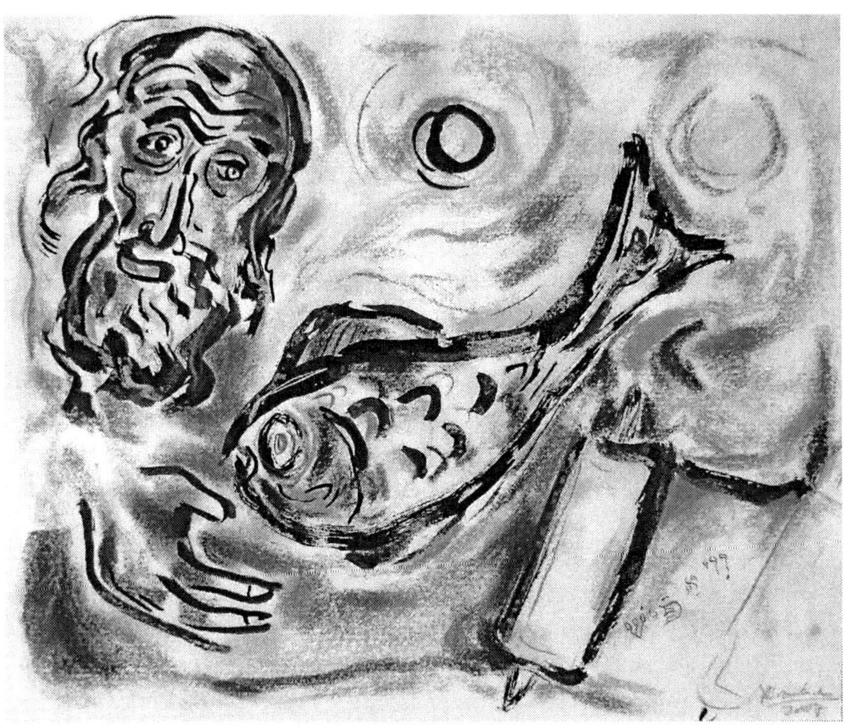

Like a Fish in Water (Vi A Fish in Vasser)

A Jew is at home in the Torah as a fish in the water. Take him out and he dies.

Inner Miracles of the Body

Alexander Tsiaras is an artist with a mission. As a child he constructed and painted the Visible Man model that showed the organs, arteries, and veins of the human body. Now he uses spectacular photographic images derived from MRI and CT scans to create anatomically correct and aesthetically beautiful pictures of the inner workings of the body that pulsate with color and life. He hopes that a ten-year rollout of images, books, and websites will inspire people to look at health and disease differently, say "Now I get it," and, most importantly, do something about their health.

Consider the extraordinary workings of the human body, trillions of cells fashioned into tissues, organs and interacting systems that provide a home for a person, alive with consciousness, capable of love. Visualize the body and consider the miracle of its design, its complexity, and its life sustaining function. See the beauty and precision of God's handiwork. In the words of the traditional prayer said upon awakening, "God formed Man in wisdom, and created within him numerous orifices and cavities."

Feel gratitude for the marvelous gift of these bodily organs that allow breathing, digestion, and movement. How can you in good faith poison them with excesses of overeating, drinking, or smoking? If you would not pour sawdust in your high-end sports car or even your old clunker, why would you pollute your body and impair its proper functioning by eating to excess?

Meditation:
I visualize the miraculous workings of the body.
I stand in awe of its complexity and beauty.
Every system harmoniously performs its function,
sustaining me and providing
a dwelling place for my soul.
Thank you, God, for bestowing upon me
this magnificent creation, my holy body.
I will honor Your creation
by keeping my body whole and healthy.
I will follow Your path of moderation and balance.
As long as my soul dwells in this body,
I will care for it lovingly and wisely.

Repeat: God, you formed the inner workings of my body with wisdom. I will cherish my body and feed it wisely.

Balance, Proportion and Harmony

Eating is both a formative and transformative act. We destroy vegetables and animals when we eat and we transform them into new substances and structures in our body. But eating can also deform as well as form. Animals are guided by instinct to eat certain foods and not others, and they limit their intake to maintain their original body form, unless overly domesticated by humans. Animals can eat as animals because they are bound by instinct that regulates their diet and food intake.

Humans are free from such instincts and, depending on culture, can eat every potential thing available. In times of plenty, we have choice over both our diet and the quantities we consume. We are even free to consume excessive amounts of food, which, at first gradually and imperceptibly, deform our body. As the external distortions develop, the internal bodily processes lose their healthy function. In extreme cases, is this not a form of indirect self-mutilation, even possibly what Karl Menninger, a renowned psychiatrist, called "partial suicide?"

But we can also choose to honor and protect the body and the good form that God intended for us. Every existing creation began as an idea in God's mind and came into being through God's will. This concept applies to both the nature of our soul and the form of our body. We can choose to pursue self-preservation and self-enhancement by maintaining the proper proportions that God had in mind when He created us. According to Kabbalah, the better we discern what God wants and bring our soul and body into alignment with God's will, the more satisfying life becomes.

Meditation:
God, You ordered the universe
with proportion and harmony,
with balance and beauty.
My body is part of this universe
and You conceived an ideal form for it,
but I strayed from the purity of Your idea.
Help me draw closer to You,
to return again to my intended state.
God, give me the strength to restore
my body to its proper form.
I will return to the path of moderation and good form.
I will engage in Holy Eating
so that I may serve you longer
with health, vigor, and energy,
with strength, devotion, and love.

Repeat: You created the universe with proportion and harmony.
Restore my body to the good form You envisioned for me.

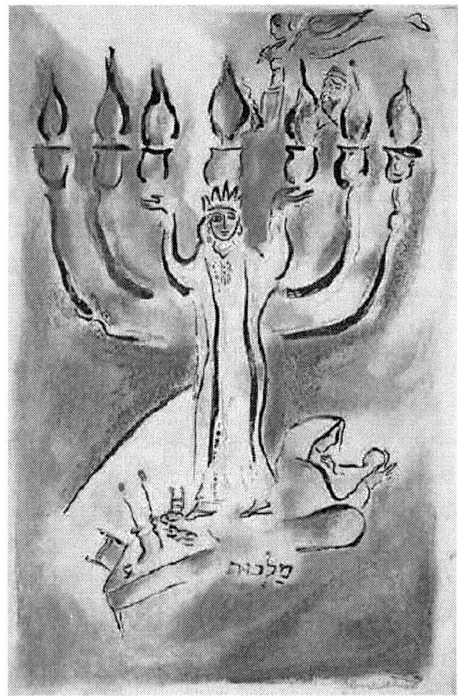

SARAH

God Loaned You this Body: Care for It

One of the first prayers upon arising expresses gratitude to God for the pure soul He has given us: "My God, the soul which you have given me is pure. You have created it, You have formed it, You have breathed it into me, and You preserve it within me...So long as the soul is within me, I offer thanks to You, Lord my God and God of my fathers, Master of all works, Lord of all souls."

Consider this same prayer with the word *body* inserted in place of *soul*: My God, the body that you have given me is pure. You have created my body, You have formed my body, and You will preserve my body. So long as my body is with me, I offer thanks to You, Lord of all souls and bodies.

In this life, the soul dwells within a body, and the body cannot exist without the soul. They are unified in the Garden of Eden but disconnected after eating from the tree of knowledge. The soul that God gave you is pure. So is the body He gave you, although it can more easily descend into impurity. The task of the human being is to maintain the purity of the soul and to elevate oneself and one's body through spiritual practices. Sadly, many continue to disconnect the body from the soul and, despite efforts to pursue otherwise great levels of spiritual perfection, neglect the body and let it be drawn down into depths of disorder and disease.

Meditation:
God, please accept these prayers
for the health of my holy soul and body.
Thank You for animating my Godly spirit
and placing it into my physical body.
You created this body and loaned it to me
until You take it from me.
While it is in my possession,
I commit to do my part to care for it.
May my Holy Eating help
to preserve its proper form,
its purity, health, and beauty.
Thank you, God,
Creator of holy souls and bodies.

Repeat: God gave me a sacred soul and body. I will care for their health and purity through Holy Eating.

I trust that through these meditations you are beginning to experience a more focused, tranquil, and inspired state of mind. I hope that you are "digesting" the concept of Holy Eating so that it is becoming as real and palpable as the physical aspects of food. Familiar biblical verses, such as "Man cannot live by bread alone" or "Taste and see that the Lord is good," will take on fresh and deeper meanings. You will understand them intimately; they will ignite your spiritual metabolism; and you will become fulfilled increasingly by the holy sparks in the food rather than by the food itself.

After you have repeated these meditations several times for the suggested 20-30 minutes, select those that are most meaningful to you and continue to rehearse them daily, or at least several times each week. Try to commit at least one entire meditation to memory, or write it on an index card that you carry with you. In addition to any blessing you normally say before and after meals, recite the meditation before you begin eating. Like any daily discipline, cultivating and maintaining this practice may be a challenge, but imagine reaping the rewards. Consider that if you eat three times or more a day, isn't it reasonable to devote at least 20 minutes of it to talking with and thanking God?

The summary statements that you repeated three to seven times at the end of each meditation are intended to engrave the message into your mind. I suggest memorizing several meditation summaries so you can draw upon them whenever you eat. At many meals or snacks, you will not have time to recite a full meditation. At the beginning of such meals, when considering second helpings, or before taking a between-meal snack, say one of the meditation summaries, preferably out loud if the setting allows. Feel free to add your own personal words or images. Remember to repeat them with *kavanah*, with spiritually connected feelings of enthusiasm, gratitude, and joy about the blessing of food that God bestows upon us with love. God is constantly thinking about and sustaining you. Keep meditating about God and your eating will be transformed.

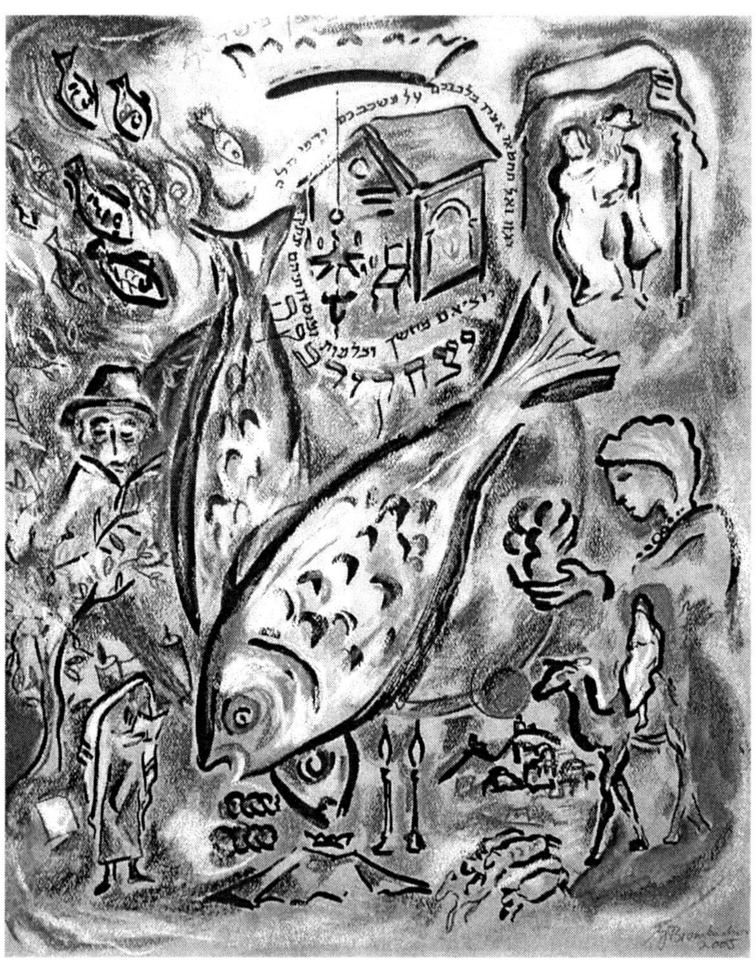

A Jewish Home

PART IV:

Not a Diet and How to Stay on It

CHAPTER 7

◆ ◆ ◆ ◆ ◆ ◆ ◆ ◆ ◆ ◆ ◆ ◆ ◆ ◆ ◆ ◆

So What Should I Eat?

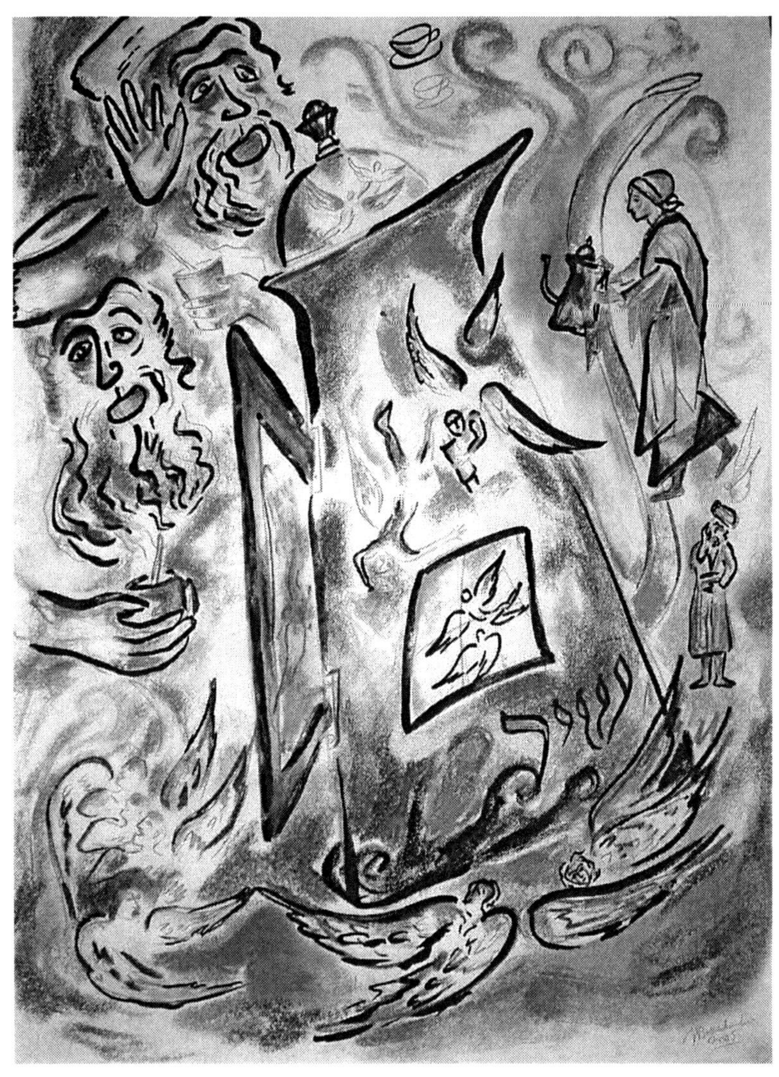

THE SINGING OF THE ANGELS

I have resisted speaking about what to eat because the strong human yearning to focus on details of eating might have distracted you from the central thesis of this book: The essence of Holy Eating is *how* you eat. As Dr. Joel Hecker, noted earlier, observes in *Mystical Bodies, Mystical Meals,* none of the kabbalistic texts describe the menus of ceremonial feasts. If the foods themselves had mattered, the texts would have mentioned them. Aside from the rules for kosher diet, the Bible does not specifically limit what foods may be eaten. Only general principles about what to eat can be extracted from biblical sources.

This may be because people should be empowered to make their own choices rather than being told what to do. This applies to eating as well. Certain individuals may react so negatively to sugar that they become addicted to it and may find that following a strictly sugar-free diet is necessary. But many who do not fall in this category prefer latitude in defining what they eat. Certainly food preferences are very personal. I recall one of my clients, a non-Jewish chef who worked in a nursing home, who learned about the particularity of food preferences through the complaints and requests that the potato latkes should be made the way each residents' mother had made them.

Holy Eating holds that God gave you intelligence so you could make free choices, and you can apply this capacity to all aspects of your life—especially eating. Many people who have tried several adequate diets know that they don't need to be told what to eat so much as how to stay with the plan. I encourage you follow the guidelines given below but as much as possible to discover what at God's banquet provides the most fulfilling food plan for you. This approach is consistent with using the consciousness that God gave you to make choices for yourself and to function more autonomously in life generally. Ask God for guidance and you will be able to determine the healthy diet that is right for you.

Today, with extensive media coverage of dieting and health information readily available on the Internet, many people who are reading this book already know quite a bit about healthy eating. If you currently have a credible food plan, stick with it but add Holy Eating to the menu. If you feel that consulting a nutritionist might give you confidence in establishing a healthy diet, it can't hurt to seek professional input. Twelve-step self-help groups provide outstanding guidance and support that is very consistent with the concepts offered here. But ultimately you will need to experiment and adjust what you eat to find the right balance of caloric input and output that empowers you to transform your weight, to maintain the new weight, and, importantly, to consistently feel contentment, joy, and even spiritual satiation through your eating.

I will offer some general guidelines derived from biblical and kabbalistic sources that can help to provide some overall structure to this stage of your journey. Since tastes and styles do vary, be creative as you forge your own path through the vast arena of culinary choices.

God Served Us Vegetation First, Meat Second

God's first diet for Man, noted earlier, included only plants. God added meat only after Noah emerged from the ark, perhaps because people were now able to accomplish the more difficult task of elevating meat. From this sequence we can infer that our primary foods should be vegetables, grains, legumes, and fruits, with meat being secondary—just the opposite of the traditional American diet, which designates meat as the main course and vegetables as the side dishes. In the past, meat was difficult to obtain, as it remains today in many parts of the world. So throughout history, the majority of humans have eaten mostly vegetarian foods, using meats only secondarily.

We can infer from God's response to the Israelites' cravings in the desert that He did not intend meat for daily consumption by humans. As noted earlier, when the Israelites complained that they missed meat in the desert, God told Moses to tell the people, "So God will give you meat and you will eat. Not for one day shall you eat, nor two days, nor five days, nor ten days, nor twenty days. Until an entire month of days, until it comes out of your nose, and becomes nauseating to you..."[64] In the modern era, eating meat daily would hardly nauseate, and until recently Americans idealized eating meat regularly. I recall that when I was growing up, a meat or chicken dish constituted the main course daily, and even during the lean college years I frequently ate steak, which sold for a mere seventy-nine cents a pound.

The biblical verses describing eating meat day after day as grinding repetition suggest that this practice was neither common nor desirable. Meat was expensive and scarce because hunting and raising animals were both so difficult. Most likely the ancients ate meat only to enhance the Sabbath table or for other religious or special occasions.

The Sages of the Talmud have said that, "A boor is forbidden to eat meat."[65] Rabbi Simon Jacobson noted[66] that the license given to Man to subjugate and consume the creatures of the world is not unconditional. Rather, it is contingent upon his sensitivity to the spiritual essence of God's creations, and his commitment to serve them by making them components of his sanctified life.

It takes an individual with broad spiritual horizons to relish a steak properly. Although today we can easily picture a crude person thoughtlessly devouring meat with lust, apparently in the days of the Talmud eating meat was restricted to the spiritually sensitive person who could sanctify the animal through his eating. Since elevated eating by such persons of "broad spiritual horizons" may not be the norm, it behooves us to be more humble and eat meat only sparingly.

In many ways the modern world is upside down, and eating more meat than vegetables is one case in point. Consistent with the biblical model and adding to the compelling research on the health hazards of red meat, a study conducted at Harvard Medical School found that women who ate meat daily had twice the risk for hormone-related breast cancer. In a diet derived from biblical principles and consistent with Holy Eating, vegetables and grains should be the main course and meat the side dish. And a fruit plate makes a wonderful dessert.

God Promised a Land of Milk and Honey, Not Refined Sugar and Flour

"I shall descend to rescue it from the hand of Egypt and to bring it up from that land to a good and spacious land, to a land flowing with milk and honey..."
—Exodus 3:8

Rabbi Moshe Loeb of Sassov (1745-1807) was well versed in both Talmud and Kabbalah. Moshe Loeb especially loved simple folks and poor or oppressed people, and was hence called the "father of widows and orphans." He loved to dance, and composed niggunim (traditional chassidic melodies).

Rabbi Moshe Loeb was not a rich man. In fact, his wife did not have enough good food for him and she could afford to make just one small pot of coffee each day. She knew her husband loved coffee more than anything and she saved up for coffee, often putting this pot in his study so that he would find it when he came home from the bayt hamidrash.

One day two Chassidim came to see the Sassover Rebbe. When they did not find him home they decided to wait in his study. They saw a nice warm pot of fresh coffee on the table and they helped themselves generously, drinking it all.

When the rebbetzin found out she was furious and she complained to her husband.

"Don't be upset', he told her, 'they didn't mean any harm. I forgive them, because those two always sing so beautifully that they open up my heart and I can hear the angels sing!"

God promised a land of milk and honey, not processed sugar and bleached flour. This is not necessarily an argument for eating only organic or natural foods. In some cases God gives us the wisdom to modify nature in healthful ways, such as by transforming mold into penicillin or milk into cheese. But as a general guideline for eating, the verse suggests that we stay close to the land and be cautious when introducing altered or processed foods into our diet.

Refined sugars are particularly difficult to include in any program of weight transformation and should be kept to an absolute minimum, if eaten at all. The Bible mentions honey but not refined sugar. Today we know that refined sugar is a "bad" carbohydrate because it has a higher glycemic index, which means it breaks down rapidly into glucose and raises blood sugar levels. This process boosts energy but also causes an insulin spike that can result in more cravings for unnecessary calories that are more likely to be stored as fat tissue. "Good" carbohydrates break down more gradually into glucose and don't raise blood sugar levels as much, providing a steadier, more stable source of energy without the cravings and weight gain.

During actual weight loss, it may be necessary to eliminate refined sugar entirely; thereafter it may be used sparingly, depending on your sensitivity to sugar addiction. I avoid sugar entirely during the week but include a sugar-based dessert at one Sabbath meal (or two if they look really good). I typically take reduced portions, such as only a half a piece of cake, rather than sample full servings of several varieties, as was my standard practice in the past. Over time I have transformed my taste sensitivities so that I don't require added sweeteners to most foods or beverages. If I desire sweets during the week, I eat only foods sweetened with fruit juices, evaporated cane juice, agave nectar or sucralose. (Sucralose, sold as Splenda, has no calories and 600 times the sweetness of refined sugar or sucrose; more than 100 studies over 20 years have shown that sucralose does not raise blood sugar levels or have toxic health effects.)

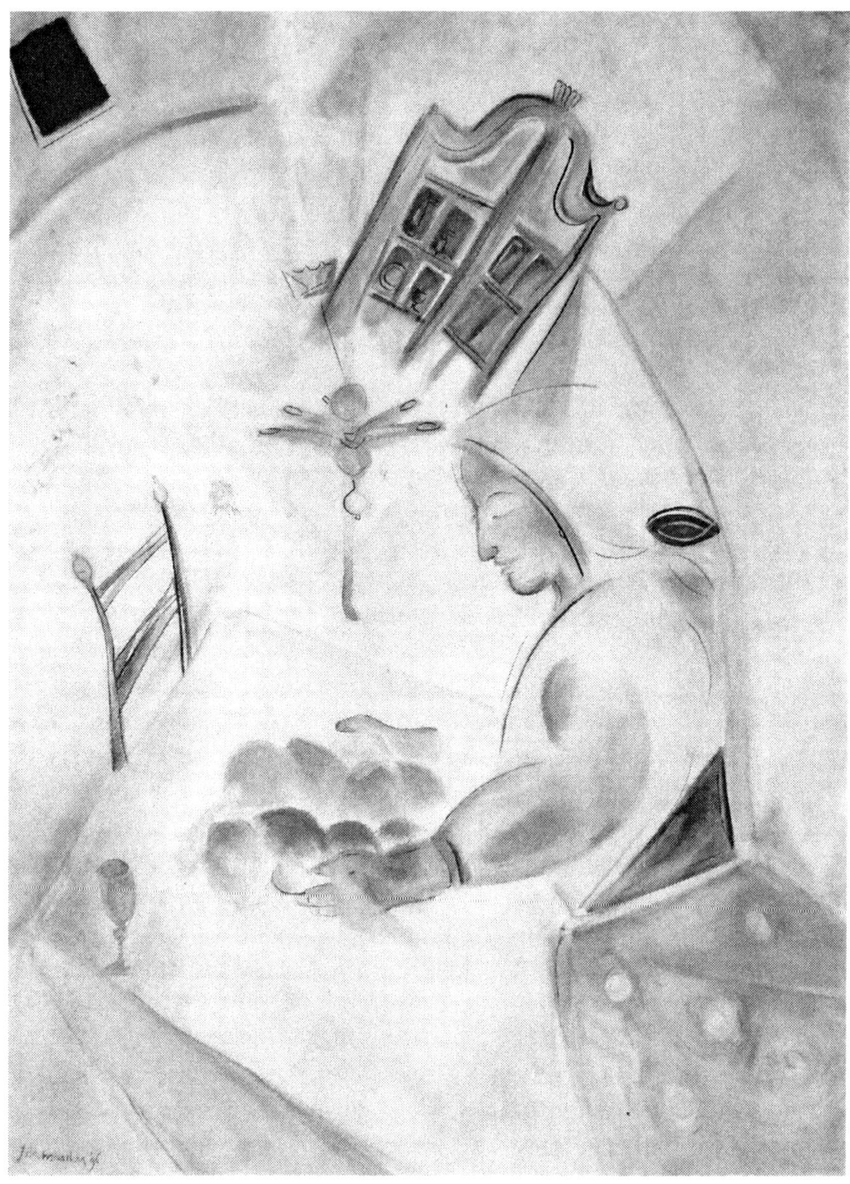

THE BERDITCHEVER RABBI'S WIFE (THE REBBETZIN)

Also to be minimized are white flour and pastas. Refined flour was not known in the biblical era. It came later and was initially hard to produce and therefore expensive. Historically, simple people ate whole-grain bread while the more affluent ate white bread. (As we have noted, the Bible warns that when Israel prospers it will become fat, and kick and rebel against God.) But as people become more health-conscious, this pattern is reversing as whole-grain products become more desirable and therefore more costly. "Good" carbohydrates, found in whole grains, beans, and nuts, can be eaten regularly, but as with any food, in moderation. I rarely eat bread during the week but will enjoy moderate portions of beautifully braided challah (egg bread) at Sabbath and holiday meals.

Caution: Drugs May Be Hazardous to Your Weight

Alcohol is a legal drug; studies have shown that it improves heart health when taken in moderation. However, the Bible demonstrates that from the earliest stage of human history, alcohol use could lead to loss of self-control and resulting shame. Once again, Noah is involved. Although he was righteous enough to have been saved from the Flood, immediately after he left the Ark, he "debased himself and planted a vineyard. He drank of the wine and became drunk, and he uncovered himself within his tent."[67]

The message to humankind is clear. Adam and Eve ate the forbidden fruit; over the next ten generations the world plunged into degeneracy and was destroyed by the Flood; and the first act of the righteous Noah was to get drunk and shame himself. We generally haven't thought of biblical history as being about eating and drinking, but they are major motifs. Although wine is used for sacramental purposes and to lighten the spirit on joyous occasions, the first message after the restoration of the world is that this drug can be dangerous and must be used in strict moderation if it is to be healthful.

Holy Eating involves limited use of alcohol for several reasons. The primary one is that alcohol diminishes conscious awareness and reduces self-control, both of which are pillars of a spiritual life and specifically of Holy Eating. Excessive alcohol consumption leads to unrestrained, gluttonous eating of unnecessary foods as well as other inappropriate behaviors. Alcohol is itself a significant source of carbohydrates and added calories—note the proverbial beer belly. You need not join the Temperance Society, but if you want to transform your weight through Holy Eating, you must use alcohol judiciously, if at all.

Research has shown that caffeine improves attention and performance while carrying no known health risks (aside from the nervous symptoms of "caffeinism" from over-use). I know of no biblical source that addresses the dangers of caffeine. But I was intrigued by Dr. Atkins, originator of the diet I previously followed, who claimed that caffeine stimulates appetite and therefore should be eliminated. Although I occasionally have a cup of caffeinated coffee or tea, I have experienced fewer food cravings and a greater sense of control over my appetite since switching almost entirely to decaffeinated drinks.

Because I Can Doesn't Mean I Should

The words quoted earlier from the Alter Rebbe imply an important Chassidic principle for living: If something is explicitly prohibited, it is forbidden, but simply because something is permitted does not make it necessary. Traditional Judaism prohibits eating non-kosher foods, so these are forbidden, but that doesn't mean that one can eat everything else without restriction.

This wisdom supports Maimonides' suggestion that we should eat considerably less food than would result in satiation. This is also consistent with the key spiritual concept of humility, which implies that we should reduce our overblown sense of self along with its greedy desires. We should strive to put more into the world than we take from it, to give much and take little. With respect to food, this means we should consume only what is necessary to be healthy and productive.

Unfortunately, even some otherwise highly spiritual people don't heed this simple but profound truth. Overeating creates many immediate and familiar signs of disharmony—including bloating, fatigue, and gastric distress—as well as the less obvious long-term danger of vulnerability to disease. The amount of food we ingest should be proportionate to our bodies' need for energy, not more or less. By eating only what is necessary we harmonize inner and external reality, our bodily needs and the food being consumed. We attain a balanced state that is respectful of the living plants or animals we are destroying. When we consume living things by necessity in a holy manner, they will promote life. But when we eat them with unholy gluttony, the consequences can be fatal.

These spiritual concepts yield an important strategy of Holy Eating, one that is gaining popularity in weight-loss programs: portion control. Even if foods are permissible by religious law and deemed healthful by nutritionists, too much of a good thing becomes a bad thing. Americans think big in many constructive ways, but the inflation in portion sizes has doomed us to an epidemic of obesity. Become more humble and modest in your food desires and be thankful that you can flourish on less.

As Rabbi Soleveitchek observed, Judaism is a very quantitative religion, specifying mathematically the rules for calculating the times of festivals, the amounts of food eaten after which blessings must be said, and the minimum amount of wine needed to sanctify the Sabbath, to cite but a few examples. The fundamental question in much of moral behavior is "How much is enough?"

We can easily extrapolate the wisdom of becoming more quantitative in the holy activity of eating.

Some people find that weighing food before eating compensates for their distorted internal perceptions about how much is enough. Inspired by the study cited earlier about smaller bowls leading to smaller portions, I have relied on visual examination of the food I dish out and, when practical, using both smaller plates and cutlery. I now eat my sugar-free breakfast mix—Kashi cereal with fresh fruit, nuts, and raisins (one of my favorite meals of the day)—with a teaspoon from a small bowl. This practice slows my eating and generates a new experience—that of wondering when I will finally get done with the meal, rather than thinking, as I used to, "Where did all the food go and can I have more?"

Lastly, research has shown that people who weigh themselves regularly lose more weight and keep it off longer than those who don't. Psychology has proven that the very act of self-monitoring an undesirable behavior reduces its frequency. Taking one's inventory and monitoring behavior are consistent with spiritual practices. For those who like feedback and data, weighing once a week—or no more than once daily—can help maintain focus and motivation. But some find weigh-ins discouraging and prefer to focus exclusively on Holy Eating itself.

Remember that all such techniques are not ends in themselves but rather means toward eating with spiritual consciousness.

A Balanced Diet

As the *Wisdom of the Fathers* teaches us, "The rich person is the one who is happy with his lot." Holy Eating can transform the idea of a "rich" meal from one that is heavy with fat into one that is balanced, not according to your inflated desires but according to your true spiritual needs.

The way of holiness is the middle way of balance and moderation. In his *Laws Concerning Character Traits*[68], Maimonides asserts that God follows the middle path in all things. Created in His image, we must strive to emulate Him. Maimonides shows how the teachings of the Bible require that we seek the mid-point between extremes of excess and deficiency in all character traits—for example, by preferring the middle path of frugality to the extremes of overspending or stinginess. (By the way, this truth did not escape the attention of sages of other traditions: Aristotle advised following "the golden mean" and Buddha "the middle path").

According to the Kabbalah, the spiritual energies of life are organized in polar extremes that must be balanced and harmonized. But the universal principle of balance applies not only to spiritual forces and character traits but also to physical reality. Our eating should not go to extremes of excess or deficiency in either quantity or type of food. Just as the mind and personality must be balanced, the body also needs a balanced mixture of fuels: Eating either excessive or insufficient quantities can be life threatening. For example, research has shown that too much fat in the diet results in clogged arteries and excess weight, but extreme deficiencies of fat can also be damaging. Moderate amounts, even of fat, are necessary to maintain health.

This spiritual principle of moderation suggests that the intended diet for humans is a balanced diet that optimally blends foods from the major food groups:

Fruits
Vegetables
Whole grains
Beans, legumes, and nuts
Meat, poultry, eggs, and fish
Dairy
Vegetable oils
Sweets

But what precise balance is best? I don't believe that we have a totally clear answer for all people, either from biblical sources or from scientific research, although some guidelines are emerging.[69]

Researchers have shown that in regions where people have greater longevity and reduced occurrences of cancer, heart disease, and other ailments, traditional foods are classified into pyramids that differ only superficially. Most of these food pyramids, including the Mediterranean, Asian, and Latin American, show that the bulk of the diet should come from fruits and vegetables or whole grains, beans, and legumes. These mainstays are supplemented by small amounts of dairy products, poultry, fish, vegetable oils, and nuts. Meat, eggs, and sweets should be consumed even less frequently.

Local crops and customs drive these pyramids' minor variations—not different ideas about nutrition. For example, the Latin American pyramid emphasizes cornmeal and tortillas, whereas the Asian includes rice and noodles. Essentially, all the pyramids are consistent with the principles extrapolated from the biblical sources. They all emphasize fruits and vegetables, minimize meat and refined sugar and flour, and recommend wine and caffeine only in moderation.

In summary, the essential food guidelines derived from the Bible and supported by contemporary food pyramids recommend the following:

- Eat more fruits, vegetables, and whole grains
- Reduce saturated fat, trans-fat, and cholesterol
- Limit sweets to a minimum
- Drink alcohol in moderation, if at all
- Control portion sizes and the total number of calories consumed
- Consider limiting or eliminating caffeine

There is nothing surprising about these general guidelines: They are as old as the Bible itself and yet remain refreshingly relevant today. But recall that research has not conclusively established the superiority of one pyramid over another and they are more similar than different. I suggest that you experiment until you find a food plan that offers you the greatest level of physical and spiritual satisfaction. But remember NOT to put the diet or food plan first, because success ultimately depends not on which foods you choose but rather on how you eat them—with or without holiness. Once you imbue a balanced diet with the attitudes of Holy Eating, then you will experience a transformation of your weight and be on the way to eternal weight loss.

CHAPTER 8

◆ ◆

Eternal Weight Loss: Keep the Focus on Faith

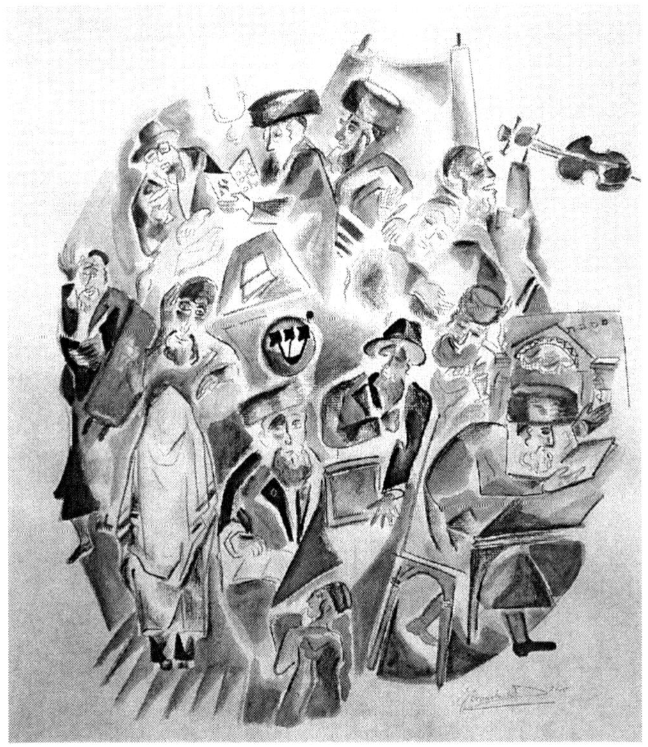

MANY PATHS

Rabbi Dov Ber of Radoschitz once asked his teacher and master, the famed "Seer of Lublin" about the right path to the service of G-d.

Answered the Seer: "There is no such thing as the right path to serve God. Because there is a path of learning, there is a path of fasting, there is a path of eating, there is a path of meditation, and so on... Also, no two persons are the same. We each have our own appropriate path to connect with the Almighty.

"But the path that you choose you must follow with all your might..."

By now some of you may have already begun Holy Eating and are successfully transforming your weight. Others may be still be reading and preparing for the stage of action. Regardless of where you are in your pursuit of Holy Eating and weight transformation, ***the key to success is establishing and maintaining focus***. The primary reason that projects of great vision fail is the inability to maintain focus. And the reason that people who have successfully reduced their weight after a monumental effort regain what they lost, is that they lost focus. If you want to sustain a program of Holy Eating, remember these three words: Focus, focus, focus.

But when the focus is primarily on the latest diet or even your personal motivation to lose weight, keeping the focus proves difficult and elusive. The problem is that diets come and go and human motivation is fleeting. Nearly every dieter has found that times of acute crisis or mounting personal stress, or even times of celebration such as holidays or vacations, can easily dismantle years of dieting success. People who rely too heavily on physical exercise to regulate their weight find that their commitment to exercise is transitory, often as fickle as the changing weather.

But God is eternal. Eternal means lasting for all time, unaffected by the passage of time or events that occur within time. By linking any sphere of life to God's will, you transcend the fluctuations of human folly and the vicissitudes of time. Recognize that God is keenly interested in how YOU eat, so much so that He established eating as humankind's first free choice to be holy or unholy. Remain connected to God and you discover the secret of eternal weight loss. No matter how great our commitment to personal goals, this commitment is finite and has limits; the extent and depth of commitment to God is infinite, without limit. Keep the focus on faith and lasting success is guaranteed.

But as we also learned from the lessons of the Garden, the serpent is wily and is always in pursuit, nipping at our heels to trip us up. The serpent patiently waits for us to turn us away from God for a split moment when we lose God-consciousness long enough to take the next fateful bite of forbidden fruit. So this chapter offers strategies derived primarily from cognitive-behavioral methods designed to maintain treatment gains and prevent relapse. Psychologists discovered that it is not enough to help people change, but we must also provide a systematic program called *relapse prevention,* a set of strategies to maintain focus over the long haul. This is especially important with eating so you can replace the endless yo-yo cycle of weight loss and weight gain with a lasting weight transformation.

Holy Eating Principles

The principles of Holy Eating can be summarized as follows:

1. Holy Eating involves eating every meal with God-consciousness rather than self-consciousness. Invite God to the table and align your will with God's will.
2. God wants you to be healthy and trim. Eat only what is necessary rather than whatever is desired.
3. Focus on the divine aspect of the food—the holy sparks. Shift from physical to spiritual metabolism and strive to experience mystical satiation.
4. Reduce the amount of food intake by 25 percent of current levels.
5. Rebalance your meals to make meat a side dish. Increase the amount of whole grains, non-trans fats, vegetables and fruits.
6. Minimize or eliminate refined sugar and refined white flour.
7. Consume alcohol and caffeine in moderation, if at all.

Keep Yourself on Your Toes: Question Your Actions

To remain focused on the Holy Eating principles, ask yourself a series of questions related to each principle. Internalize these questions so that you can focus on them as you develop your food plan and pose one or more of them to yourself before each meal or snack. The primary questions, "Am I eating with holiness?" and "Does God want me to eat this?" should be stated every time you eat.

Questions:

1. Eat every meal with God-consciousness rather than self-consciousness. Align your self and body with God's will.

    Am I eating with holiness?
    Does God want me to eat this?
    Am I eating to serve God or my own selfish pleasure?
    Do I feel connected to God at this moment?
    Have I said a blessing or thanked God for the food?

2. Eat only what is necessary rather than whatever is desired.

    Even though this is permitted on my meal plan, is it necessary?
    Do I need to eat this or is it just indulgence?
    Is this true appetite for food or for something else that is missing in life?

3. Focus on the divine aspect of the food—the holy sparks. Shift from physical to spiritual metabolism and strive to feel mystical satiation.

    Am I looking beyond the physical food to see that it comes from God?
    Do I taste God's nourishing love in the food He provides for me?
    Have I paused to feel God's warm light that fulfills me constantly?
    Am I eating as a service to God?

4. Reduce the amount of food intake by 25 percent of current levels.

    Have I thought about the portion size before serving the food?
    Did I measure the food visually or with a scale to make sure my eyes don't deceive?
    Have I thought that retraining impulses by eating less pleases God?
    Did I pause during the meal and leave some food over?

5. Minimize or eliminate refined sugar and refined white flour.

    Have I established a clear plan to eliminate all sugar or allow sugar only on the Sabbath or special occasions?
    Do I have adequate substitute sweeteners?
    Have I focused on sweetening the meal spiritually?

6. Rebalance your meals to make meat more of a side dish. Increase the amount of grains and vegetables.

   Do I really need a 10-ounce steak or can I be satisfied with 1/2 that amount?
   What does the Bible say about the dangers of craving meat?
   Have I served the meal with meat as a side dish rather than main course?
   Am I eating meat with proper reverence that will elevate it?

7. Eat each meal with a sense of gratitude to God for providing abundantly and caring for all your needs.

   Did I say a blessing before eating with concentration and sincerity?
   Did I connect with God and thank Him for His loving kindness?
   Did I say grace after meals or thank God for satisfying my appetite?

Mood and Food

"You have turned my mourning into dancing; You have loosened [the cords of] my sackcloth and girded me with joy."
—Psalm 30:11—

Once the concept of Holy Eating is fully embraced with deep belief, engraved into the mind and locked onto, weight transformation can become both simple and easy. The challenging part is keeping the faith alive so it penetrates your consciousness and influences your behavior consistently. Every life is replete with ups and downs, emotional hassles of everyday living and major crises that can evoke anxiety, sadness, anger, isolation and fatigue.

If these emotions become chronic or debilitating, treatment with psychotherapy or medication may be necessary for success in meeting any life task, especially changing one's relationship to food. Although we can't deal with this extensively, we must note that traumatic life events and negative moods can sometimes turn people away from God. Even the smallest upset such as an argument with a friend or spouse will provoke some to eat excessively.

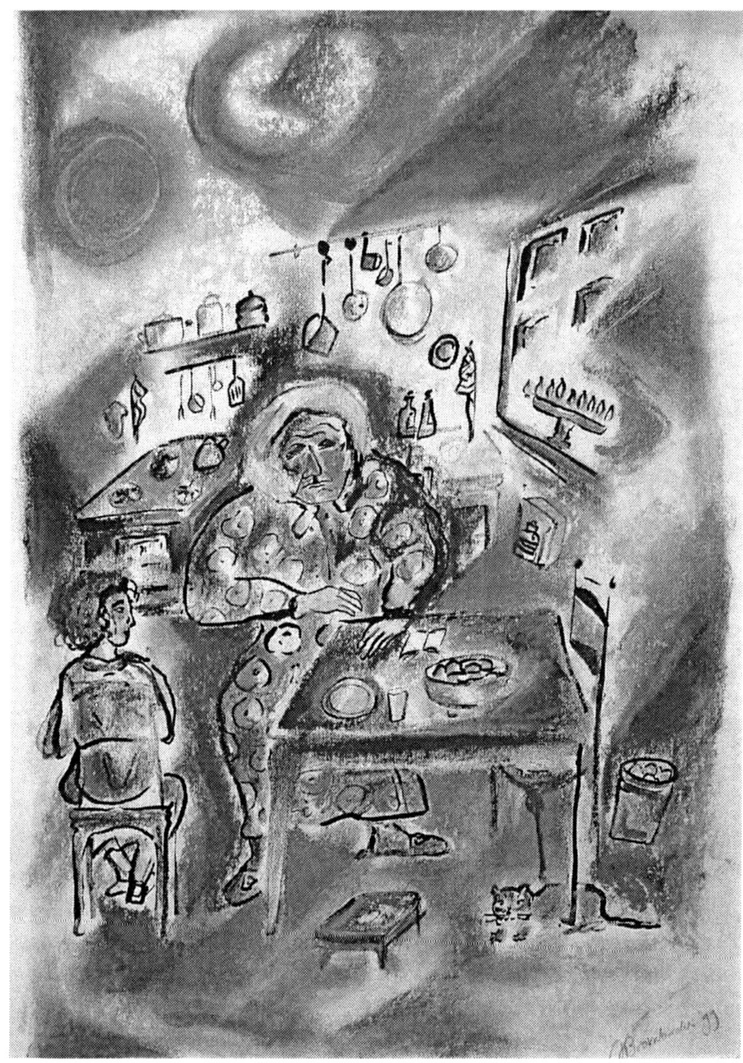

In Grandmother's Kitchen

A woman moving with increasing momentum on a spiritual path who is blindsided with a tragic loss such as the death of child may feel betrayed by God and filled with anger towards Him. Overwhelmed with anger and grief, she may turn away from God. Whether a minor irritation or a devastating loss, some degree of sadness, anxiety, anger, isolation and fatigue may occur. If these states of mind and mood cause a distance from God, the motivation to be holy and to sustain Holy Eating will be lost.

But suffering can also lead a person to turn towards God as seen in the classic spiritual transformations of addicts only after they hit "rock bottom." From a spiritual perspective, these negative states must instead become spurs to turn towards God for solace, comfort and ultimately for the transformation of the suffering into joy, the darkness into light. However remote this may feel at the moment, true faith offers the unfailing optimism that a person's suffering has a constructive purpose that transcends our current understanding and that one will find the good in every bad situation. The bad times will be followed by better days. Many volumes have been written about coping with suffering from both spiritual and psychological perspectives and the reader is advised to consult these if you are experiencing severe distress of this sort.

From the perspective of Holy Eating, the task is to elevate even these negative moods into greater closeness with God, even if this is at first through arguing and expressing open anger. Face your pain and do not turn away from God. Remain always connected and you will find solace and answers. This is the faith perspective. Remind yourself of the basic premise that the first primordial act of holiness is how Adam and Eve ate and your first response to distress may be to lash out with unholy Eating. But you can reframe your distress as an opportunity to remain on the path of holiness by re-affirming that food is not the answer to negative emotion, pain or suffering. Love of God and staying connected to holiness despite negative feelings is the goal. You have an opportunity at least three times daily to win this struggle. In fact, as you discover that you can even manage these times of sorrow without eating excessively, your love of God and belief in God's transforming power will grow.

A useful acronym can help you remember the mood triggers that lead people to engage in addictive behaviors: SHALT. People in self-help groups employ many cognitive-behavioral strategies and aphorisms to stay focused on controlling impulses. The term "HALT" is used in 12-step groups to remember mood states that can trigger addictive behavior: Hungry, Angry, Lonely or Tired. I have expanded this to 'SHALT' to provide an 'S' that signifies Sad. Also, I have expanded the 'A' to include Anxious as well as Anger. So we now have:

S = Sad
H = Hungry
A = Anxious and Angry
L = Lonely
T = Tired

When you feel these trigger emotions, instead of eating first repeat the words of the prayer: "Thou shalt love the Lord your God with all your heart, with all your soul and with all your might."[70] In this context, "with all your heart" can mean to love God with the negative emotions in your heart, as well as the joyful ones; "with all your soul" means to transcend beyond your personal feelings which are always divided into negatives and positives to the soul level where the distinction between negative and positive is lost in a higher unity of absolute goodness; "with all your might" returns to the human level and means you should use all your personal strength and physical resources to do God's will.

As you can see, once you succeed at overcoming negative moods and events in this way, you have transformed the eating triggers of negative moods into the holy state of Thou SHALT love the Lord your God. In effect, you have engaged in true spiritual metabolism because you have taken the energy of your negative moods and transformed them into love and connection to God. This is the dynamic that underlies the familiar experience of anyone who has found that suffering brought him closer to God rather than leading him away. When you eat with holiness whether joyful or sad, you have moved towards eternal weight transformation. Thou shalt eat with holiness.

The psalm cited at the beginning of this section contains a beautiful allusion to the transformation process that occurs when one faces sorrow by turning towards God rather than moving away. The verse does not express gratitude to God for simply removing the suffering and now giving happiness; it says that God actually turned or transformed the suffering into joy: "You turned my mourning into dancing." Similarly, the cord or belt securing the sackcloth, the coarse fabric worn by mourners, now girds me with joy. "Gird" means to secure something to oneself or to another using a belt or strap. The implication is that rather than merely "clothing" me in joy, because the person faced her suffering with faith, God will go a further step and transform the very suffering into joy and securely attach this joy to her so it will be lasting. Darkness is thus transformed into light. Weight transformation becomes steady and lasting.

Lapse, Relapse and Repentance

God made us with infinite potential for greatness, but with multiple opportunities for error. Regulating eating is challenging because one cannot practice complete abstinence as with alcohol or drug addictions and in fact must engage in eating numerous times daily. The possibilities for failure abound. In pursuit of Holy Eating, hope for success, but expect to make mistakes along the way. Slips will occur and every slip poses a threat to maintaining focus. When people feel they have relapsed, they often feel guilt, loss of self-esteem and a tendency to give up—what psychologists call the "*abstinence violation effect*."

When a slip occurs it is useful to think of this not as a *relapse* which signifies a complete failure and a full-blown slip back to where you first began. Instead, view the slip as a *lapse* in an ongoing lifelong plan that is bound to have occasional imperfections along the way. No improvement can be graphed as a straight line of progress but will always have ups and down. Progress in human tasks is more of a cyclical pattern of change that gradually moves less far and less frequently downward, but never without some fluctuations in the wrong direction.

The distinction between lapse and relapse can be related to the spiritual concept of repentance. God knows we will have lapses and has provided for this human weakness by creating the corrective path of repentance. When one deviates from the proper path, guilt is the emotion that signals that we have not lived up to an inner standard. Although lapses and guilt are inevitable, excessive guilt associated with relapses is not. Instead of beating yourself up with guilt, read the guilt as a signal and motivation to return to God, to close the gap created by unholy eating.

Repentance involves admitting an error without qualification, feeling remorse about it and committing to try to not make the same mistake again. Once you have done this, there is no longer need for guilt which has served its purpose. Most people make the mistake of misunderstanding the function of healthy guilt and either overdo it or go to the opposite extreme of wanting to have nothing to do with any guilt. Guilt management is important to the pursuit of holiness in general and to Holy Eating in particular.

There is a positive side to guilt. God is always waiting on the other side of guilt to welcome you back to the path of holiness. If fact, our Sages teach us that the one who returns to God after losing his way can reach a higher level of holiness than someone who has lived a pure and saintly life throughout. This is because through true repentance even the unholy and dark deeds become elevated into positives, thus resulting in a net gain in goodness. Don't use this as an excuse to run out and engage in unholy behavior in order to then repent because it doesn't work if you deviate with that intention. But any sincere mistake can be elevated by a sincere admission of wrong and desire to get back on track.

So when you slip, label it as a lapse and manage your guilt to feel just the right amount in order to return to God and towards Holy Eating. Let the balanced guilt—not too much or too little— become a conduit reconnecting you to God. Transform the lapse into a positive re-affirmation of your purpose to serve God in the future.

Ritual and Remembering

Rabbi Dr. Abraham Twerski noted that because a spiritual void is at the core of addictions, 12-step programs that focus on building spirituality are very successful. One can be spiritual, according to Dr. Twerski, without being religious. What do we mean, though, by spiritual and religious?

Spirituality is an attitude or outlook oriented towards the non-corporeal or spirit world rather than the physical. Interestingly, the Latin origin of the term "religion" is *re-ligare* with the root 'lig' meaning to bind or tie. Thus, religion is re-binding or connecting oneself to God or the spiritual world. Religion without spirituality would be meaningless unless used in the generalized sense of doing something, such as reading the newspaper or eating breakfast, "religiously." However, spirituality without religion can become transitory and unstable because it lacks the 'binding' aspect provided by the force of commandment and ritual that anchors the spiritual practices.

God-consciousness requires conscious awareness or else the mind will shift focus back to the self. But God has also given us the gift of forgetting which can be useful to erase the many painful and negative experiences that color every human life. The problem is that we often forget that which we should remember. Religion with its ritual practices helps us to remember to keep the faith and focus on our spiritual dimension, to keep us striving towards holiness.

To achieve eternal weight transformation, Holy Eating must be practiced religiously. Clearly from the above considerations, a set of formal "re-ligious" rituals that "bind" one to a spiritual outlook towards eating will be helpful. If we are motivated only by self-oriented desires to take off pounds, we may lose weight today only to regain it tomorrow when our attitude or mood changes. But if we believe that we are commanded to be healthy and have rituals to reinforce these commands, we will remain constant in our motivation as long as we remain true to our faith. A major concept of this book has been that regardless of your starting level of spirituality or religious practices, your daily eating regimen can become a ladder to climb towards increased holiness. Eating can become an opportunity to become more religious in the sense of re-binding yourself to God.

Many of the strategies discussed throughout this book are rooted in rituals practiced by the religiously observant: daily prayer, washing the hands, blessings said before eating, speaking words of holiness at meals, saying grace after meals. Frequently, these can drift into religious rituals without their original spiritual connection in which case they don't contribute to Holy Eating. Empty rituals during eating can result in full plates with corresponding weight gain. By linking the rituals back to the spiritual roots we achieve the essential goal of religion that is to re-bind us to the spirit world and to God.

In addition to the spiritual rituals, many people adopt behavioral strategies to help stay focused such as weighing foods, weighing themselves, counting calories, reporting meal plans and eating the same menu on a regular basis to reduce decision making, to name several common ones. These are extremely helpful for many people and, if approached in a balanced way, are consistent with spiritual eating.

But I will add a word of caution that it is important to keep these useful techniques that focus on the physical aspects of eating in perspective so that the spiritual dimension of Holy Eating remains the primary focus. The human mind tends towards the physical and the concrete. It is easier in the short run to stay in the physical world than to ascend to the spiritual. So it can be tempting to get more involved with weighing oneself or counting calories than to remain focused on eating as a spiritual service.

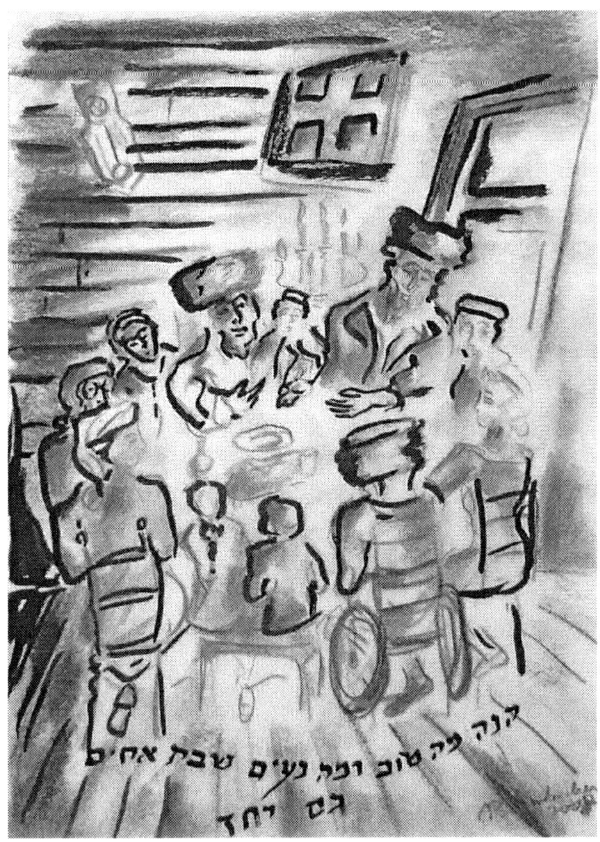

THE SHABBOS TABLE

I recall reading a recent psychological study by Dr. Rena Wing, a former colleague, published in the New England Journal of Medicine, which found more weight loss for people who frequently weighed themselves as part of the program. Intrigued by this apparent breakthrough I shifted from weekly weighing before each Sabbath to daily weighing. When I noticed with alarm that my weight could fluctuate by 3-4 pounds a day depending on the time of day I weighed myself, I felt compelled to start weighing myself several times a day. During this experiment, I realized that my attention started to drift towards the physical outcome of my eating and consequently away from how I was eating, from the essential concepts and practices of Holy Eating. So, maintain those physical rituals that are working for you, but don't make them into idols that distract you from the higher purpose of your mission.

The most useful rituals are those that serve as direct reminders of the essential concept of Holy Eating: "You shall be holy, because I, the Lord your God, am holy." Build the practices suggested in Chapters 3 and 4 into your daily eating routines and you will strengthen your attachment to Holy Eating. Write your favorite prayer on an index card and carry it with you to be read at each meal. Put a small sign on your refrigerator or dinner table with a biblical verse or short prayer that reminds you of Holy Eating and God's loving wish for you to be healthy. Keep a prayer book or book with spiritual readings near your table so you can read a short passage from it during meals. Write the questions listed earlier on a card so that you can have them available at each meal.

When it comes to control over impulses such as eating, the human mind is weak and previously learned lessons can be easily forgotten or ignored. Our Sages taught that new knowledge cannot be fully acquired until it is learned 100 times and so prescribed learning new material 101 times to guarantee it is retained. In the Wisdom of Our Fathers, we are advised regarding biblical knowledge: "Learn it and learn it, for everything is in it; look deeply into it; grow old and gray over it, and do not stir from it, for there is nothing more edifying for you than it."[71]

Our spiritual journey began with food temptations faced by Adam and Eve and by our ancestors during their many wanderings. Today we face the same struggle and it is easier than ever to lose our way. God knew that our ability to elevate eating was a vital first step towards transcending the physical as well as a symbol of our more general relationship with the material world. Holy Eating brings together the spiritual concepts and psychological tools needed to make our table into an altar, to make our body a true vessel for Godliness, and to accomplish the eternal transformation of our excess weight into positive energy and acts of loving-kindness.

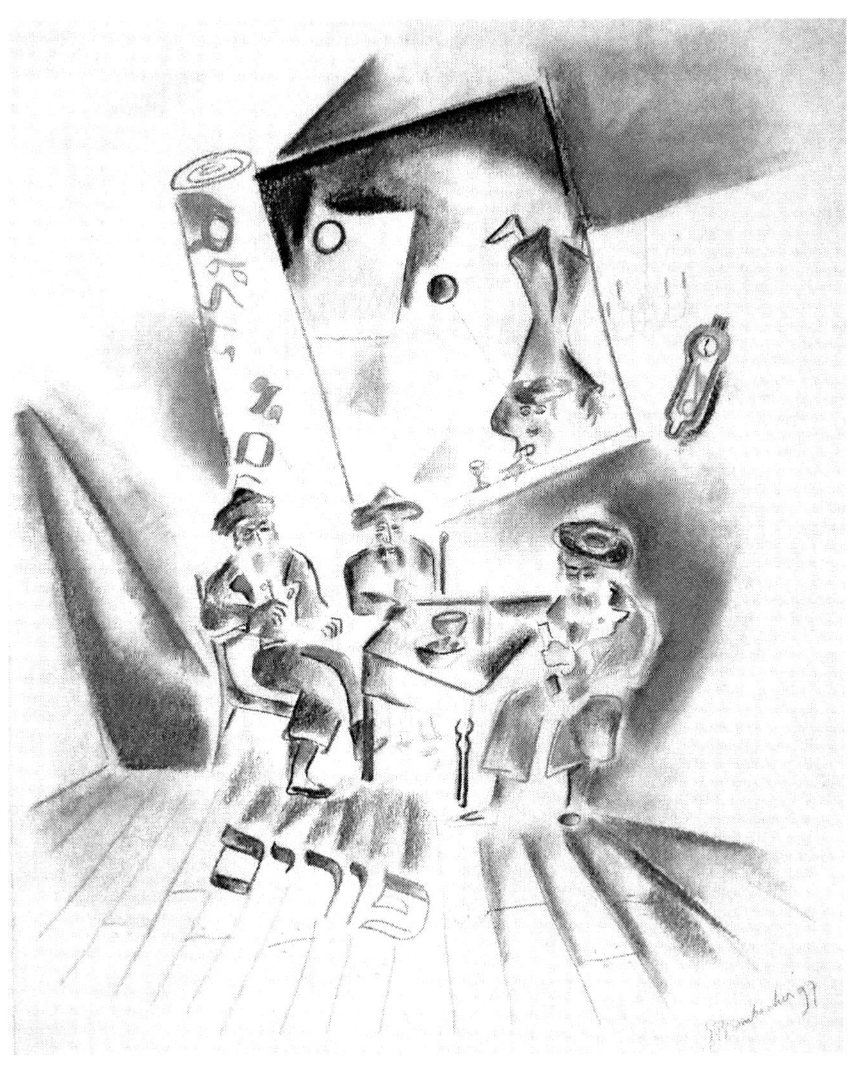

Purim Seudah (Purim Meal)

Glossary

Aliyah: Literally means ascent or going up, but commonly used in the context of moving to the state of Israel or being called to read from the Torah during religious services.

Alter Rebbe: Rabbi Schneur Zalman of Liadi *(1745-181),* originator of the Chabad Chassidic movement and author of the Tanya.

Baal Shem Tov: Rabbi Yisroel ben Eliezer (1698-1760), Jewish mystic and founder of the Chassidic movement, who emphasized rapturous prayer and joyful celebration.

Binah: The spiritual energy posited by the Kabbalah that generates the intellectual faculty of the mind corresponding to developing a detailed understanding or comprehension of an idea.

Chabad Lubavitch: Popular branch of Chassidic Judaism originated by Rabbi Schneur Zalman of Liadi, the Alter Rebbe, in the late 1700s. Chabad stands for the emphasis placed on the intellectual faculties of Chochmah (Wisdom or Conception), Binah (Understanding or Contemplation) and Daas (Intimate Knowledge).

Chassidism: Spiritual revival movement initiated in the 18th century by Rabbi Israel Baal Shem Tov at a time when Jewry was devastated by Cossacks, false messianism and poverty. In addition to learning the Torah laws, Chassidic philosophy emphasizes meditating on God's greatness and on the inner significance of the commandments and rituals. Such contemplation is intended to further refine one's character and interpersonal relations, to enhance the joyful observance of the commandments and ultimately to hasten the coming of the Messianic Era.

Chochmah: The spiritual energy posited by the Kabbalah that generates the intellectual faculty of the mind corresponding to the initial spark or conception of an idea.

Daas: The spiritual energy posited by the Kabbalah that generates the intellectual faculty of the mind corresponding to the experiential and intimate knowledge of an idea.

Devekus: Attachment to God, from the root meaning "to cling."

Kabbalah: Extensive body of Jewish mystical teachings about the nature of divinity, the creation, the soul and the role of human beings, as well as meditative, devotional and mystical practices. The term Kabbalah is derived from the root "to receive" or "to accept" and often used synonymously with "tradition".

Korbonos: Typically termed "sacrifices", but more properly considered "offerings" of grain, fruit, or animals brought to the Temple.

Maimonides, Rabbi Moshe ben Maimon*:* 12th century rabbi, physician and philosopher living in Spain, Morocco and Egypt who wrote the renowned Mishneh Torah that includes commentaries on Jewish laws pertaining to health and eating.

Manna: Food provided by God to the Israelites in the desert that had the luster of crystal and tasted like delicate cakes or took on whatever taste the person desired.

Maggid: East European Jewish religious itinerant preacher, with skill as a narrator of religious stories.

Mishneh Torah: Fourteen-volume code of Jewish law compiled in Egypt in the 12th century C.E. by Maimonides.

Nachash: Hebrew word for serpent derived from the root word meaning blind, impulsive urge, as in instinctive drive.

Olah: Elevation offering or sacrifice that stays on the flame of the Altar all night until morning and is intended to atone for impure thoughts.

Pirke Avot: Ethics of the Fathers, a collection of sayings and aphorisms about proper ethical and social behavior, compiled around the 3rd century C.E. from the Talmudic commentaries on the Bible.

Rambam: Acronym for Maimonides

Rashi: The outstanding Biblical commentator of the Middle Ages, born in Troyes, France, and living from 1040 to 1105. He wrote the authoritative commentaries on the Bible and Talmud.

Rebbe: A term for Rabbi or teacher that is used by Chassidic groups who maintain an intense and intimate relationship with their leader.

Schulchan Aruch: Code of Jewish Law that organized the complex set of biblical laws first compiled in the 16th century by Josef Karo.

Succah: Impermanent booth or tabernacle covered with cut branches from living trees in which Jews were instructed to dwell for seven days to commemorate the exodus from Egypt and thanksgiving for the harvest.

Talmud: Collection of extensive written commentaries on the Bible that record Rabbinic discussions pertaining to Jewish law, customs and history. Comprised of the Mishnah, which is the first written compendium of Judaism's Oral Law, compiled in 200 B.C. by Rabbi Judah HaNasi, and the Gemara, a detailed discussion of the Mishnah and related writings.

Tanya: 18th century book of spiritual teachings derived from Kabbalah by Rabbi Schneur Zalman of Liadi, the Alter Rebbe.

Tikkun: Concept of "repairing the world" derived from the kabbalistic belief that at the time of creation the world was shattered into shards and the task of humankind is to heal or repair the world through good deeds.

Tish: Yiddish for "table," referring to the festive meal conducted by a Chassidic Rebbe and his followers accompanied by religious speeches and enthusiastic songs.

Torah: The first five books of the Bible given to Moses by God on Mt. Sinai, including Genesis, Exodus, Leviticus, Numbers and Deuteronomy. The term Torah derives from the root "teaching", "instruction" or "law".

Yaakov Yitzchak Horowitz: (1745-1815), known as the Seer of Lublin because of his great intuitive powers.

Yeshurun: from the Hebrew word "yesher" which means straightness or uprightness and is used to remind Israel to be true to its moral calling.

Zohar: Considered one of the most important books on Kabbalah or Jewish mysticism, it was published in Spain by Moses de Leon during the 13th century C.E., although he attributed it to 2nd century C.E. Rabbi Simeon bar Yochai. The term Zohar is derived from the root "radiance" or "splendor".

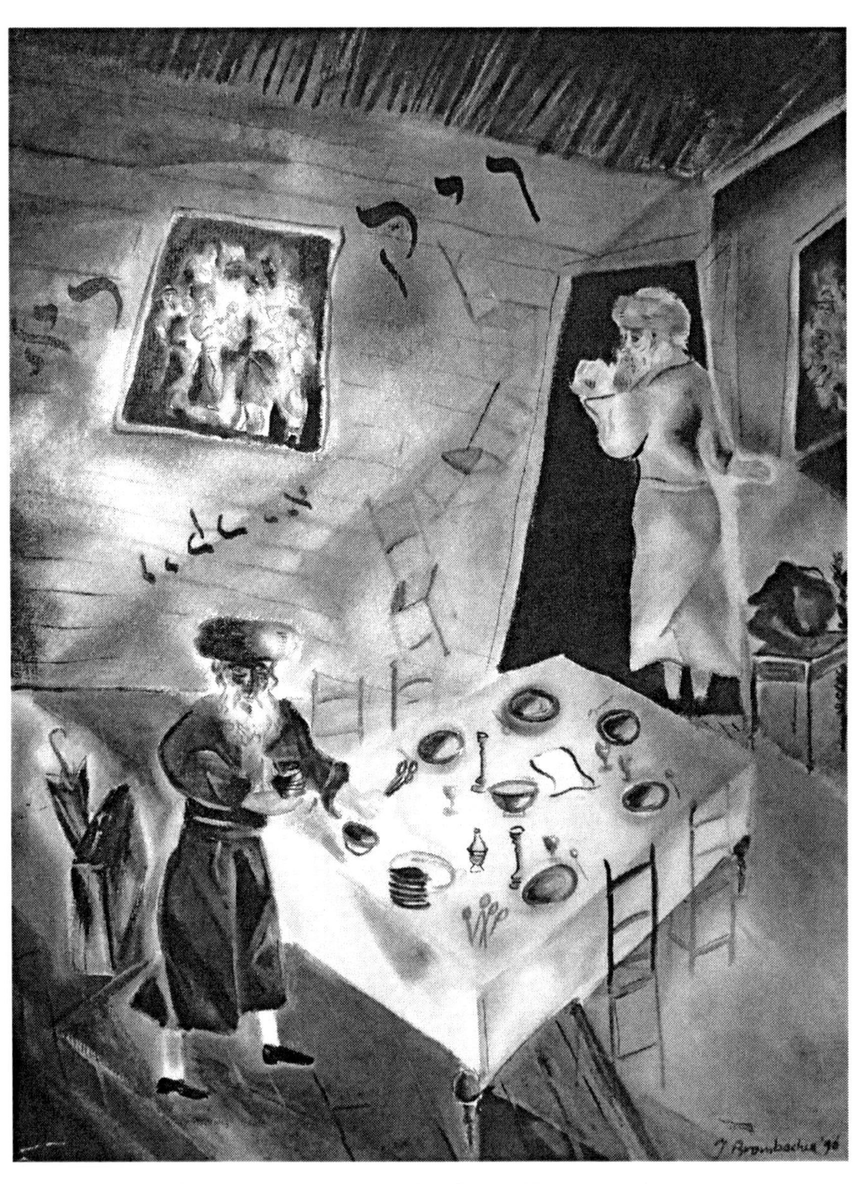

Avraham Avinu and The Besht (Abraham Our Father and The Baal Shem Tov)

Notes

1. Deuteronomy 31:20.
2. Genesis 2:7.
3. Talmud Taanit 22b.
4. Deuteronomy 4:15.
5. Deuteronomy 7:15.
6. Leviticus Rabbah 16:8.
7. Holy Eating: Insights Into Tu B'Shevat, Chabad.org.
8. Rabbi Tsadok and other scholars, by the way, believe the forbidden fruit was not an apple but a fig. If *what* Adam and Eve had eaten was more important than *how*, no doubt figs, or apples, would be prohibited today. The Bible forbids many foods, but the literal forbidden fruit is not one of them.
9. Genesis: 1:29-31
10. Genesis 8: 3-4.
11. Rabbi Horowitz (the Shelah).
12. Shnei Luchos HaBris.
13. Genesis 25:29.
14. Numbers 11:4-6.
15. Psalm 107:5-7.
16. Numbers 11:20.
17. Kibroth-hattaavah.
18. Numbers 11: 33-34.
19. Deuteronomy 32: 15
20. Hirsch, 1986, 804-805.
21. Exodus 15:2 & 15:11.
22. Exodus 16:3.
23. Exodus 16:4.
24. Rabbi Eliezer Hamudai.
25. Pesachim 118a.
26. Exodus 24:10-11.
27. Rashi and Maimonides.
28. Rabbi Yehudah, quoted in the Zohar.
29. Shulchan Aruch 231:1.
30. Mishneh Torah, Hilchos Deos 3:2.

31. Talmud, Kiddushin 40b.
32. Hilchos Deos 4:1.
33. Hilchos Deos 4:2.
34. Although these assertions follow logically from the Biblical texts and the writings of Maimonides, they cannot be applied without further information to a given individual. There are medical conditions such as Prodder-Willy Syndrome, for example, in which the hunger center in the brain does not provide normal signals of satiation. Such an individual will continue to eat to excess because he or she does not get cues that their hunger is satisfied.
35. Rebbe Schneur Zalman (1745-1812), founder and first rabbi of Chabad Chassidism, was the author of many works including the *Schulchan Aruch HaRav* and the *Tanya*, which earned him the designation Baal HaTanya. He was the prominent disciple of the Maggid of Mezeritch, who in turn was the successor of the founder of Chassidism, the Baal Shem Tov.
36. The Complete Artscroll Siddur, p. 15.
37. Based on the teachings of Rabbi Menachem Mendel Schneerson, renowned 20th century leader of the Chabad movement.
38. Exodus 25:8.
39. Exodus 15:2.
40. Keter Shem Tove: Teaching 194.
41. Reshit Hochmah Sh'ar ha-Kedushah, as quoted in Buxbaum, p. 235.
42. Rabbi Elimelech of Lizensk
43. Mazkeret Shem ha-Gedolim, p. 43, as quoted in Buxbaum, 1990, p. 226.
44. Likutey Moharan II, 16.
45. Perceived food hunger can also be lack of hydration, in which case drinking water or a non-caloric beverage can satisfy the need.
46. Research conducted at Harvard Medical School found that over time fewer families have been eating together and that eating family meals was associated with more healthful dietary intake. A National Survey of Children's Health from the Center for Disease Control reports that in 2003 only 42 percent of adolescents aged 12 to 17 ate a meal with their family 6 to 7 times per week. Thirty-one percent had 0 to 3 family meals. A study conducted at Columbia University found that the more often children had dinner with their parents, the less likely they were to drink, smoke, or use illegal drugs.

47. Rabbi Levi Yitzhak of Berditchev , Ohalei Shem, p. 26, #45, as quoted in Buxbaum, 1990, p. 227.
48. Ezekiel 41:22.
49. Rabbi Yeheil Michal, cited in Buxbaum, 1990, p. 238.
50. Grace After Meals.
51. Exodus 16:20.
52. Exodus 16:24.
53. Cited in Buxbaum, 1990, p. 257.
54. See Buxbaum, 1990.
55. Psalm 34: 9-11.
56. Psalm 40: 9.
57. Exodus 34:28.
58. Deuteronomy 8:10.
59. Kezayit
60. Exodus 16: 16-18.
61. Wineberg, 1987, 362.
62. Rabbi Aharon Perlov of Karlin (1736-1772), "HaGadol," the author of Avodas Yisroel and several homiletical works on the Zohar and Psalms.
63. See his excellent books, such as *Jewish Meditation*, *Meditation and the Bible*, and *Meditation and Kabbalah.*
64. Numbers 11:18-20.
65. Talmud, Pesachim 49b.
66. Based on the teachings of the Rabbi Menachem Mendel Schneerson.
67. Genesis 9:20-21.
68. *Hilkhos De'os.*
69. You can find a useful comparison of different food pyramids at the Mayo Clinic's web site (www.mayoclinic.com) or go directly to http://www.mayoclinic.com/health/healthy-diet/NU00190.
70. Deuteronomy 10:12.
71. Pirke Avos 5:21

Acknowledgments

Writing a book is a challenging task. Completely identifying all the positive influences that helped bring it to fruition is impossible. Even my scientific writings have seemed more like a gift from God than a personal accomplishment. How much more so with this work, that is a summary of the spiritual truths of biblical and chassidic wisdom applied to the daily act of eating. I am grateful to Hashem for the mysterious forces that empowered these spiritual ideas to literally transform my flesh and for the opportunity to share this with others. I also wish to thank all the teachers, friends and associates who have taught me directly and indirectly, inspired and challenged me, lifted my spirits and made me laugh—all valued contributors to this work.

On a more down to earth level, there are also some individuals who merit personal acknowledgement. I am especially grateful to my wife, Amy, who is an inspiring role model for living a spiritually oriented life directed towards self-discovery and improvement. Thank you for reading several drafts of the manuscripts, for your consistent encouragement and occasional, lovingly delivered messages that this book *will* be completed. Her presence in this book is manifest both in the content and between the lines.

For the past 20 years, Rabbi Yosef Rosenblum has been a valued friend, gifted teacher, inspirational model of a well-lived life—and even an occasional biking partner. Thank you for providing general affirmation of the religious content that gave me the confidence to complete the work. Any inaccuracies in the text or incorrect interpretations of the sources are of course my own.

I enjoyed and appreciated many Sabbath meetings with Rabbi Mordechai Rosenberg during which we learned Jewish concepts related to food and eating. Rabbi Yudel Huberman served as a scholarly research assistant who helped track down Talmudic and Chassidic sources related to the topic. Rabbi Sholom Cohen, Richard Busch and Joan Polzin read and provided helpful comments on the manuscript. A special thanks to Rabbi Yosef Silverman who, after hearing my ideas, suggested that I write this book.

I benefited from the professional editing of Steve Levin, formerly of the Pittsburgh Post-Gazette, whose challenging critiques helped sharpen the focus and bring the, at times, lofty ideas to a practical level. Judith Sanders served as a "writing coach" whose enthusiasm about the book ensured its completion and as an editor, added graceful touches to the style of expression.

Several "trusted servants" of Overeaters Anonymous International were willing to share their stories of how they used spiritual principles to successfully lose weight.

Lastly, I am grateful to the participants of my workshops on Holy Eating who, in implementing these ideas, furthered my understanding of both the power and struggles of pursuing a spiritually based path to health and weight transformation.

About the Author

Robert M. Schwartz, Ph.D. is an internationally recognized clinical psychologist who has published dozens of scientific papers on positive thinking, emotional wellbeing and successful behavior change. He has written popular articles and op-ed pieces for national newspapers such as *The Week: The Best of U.S. and International Media, The Christian Science Monitor, Pittsburgh Post-Gazette* and *The Jewish Chronicle.*

Dr. Schwartz is President and Founder of Cognitive Dynamic Therapy Associates, a multi-specialty psychological group practice employing 10 therapists. He is also Adjunct Assistant Professor of Psychiatry at the University of Pittsburgh School of Medicine where he teaches psychiatry residents and conducts research on positive thinking, emotional balance and mental health.

For over 30 years, Dr. Schwartz has specialized in cognitive approaches to behavior change, with an emphasis on mood disorders, health behaviors and addictions. For the past 20 years he has studied Jewish spirituality and Chassidic philosophy. He and his wife live in Pittsburgh, Pennsylvania and Atlanta, Georgia. They have seven sons between them. Correspondence to Dr. Schwartz can be sent to *robsch77@gmail.com.*

About the Illustrator

Shoshannah Brombacher, Ph.D. is an author/artist and trained storyteller from Amsterdam, who taught and studied Medieval Hebrew literature and more at the Universities of Leyden, Berlin and Jerusalem. She currently lives in Brooklyn, NY with her family. Her art is inspired by the teachings of Chassidic Masters, which fascinated her since she found them in her father's study long ago. Dr. Brombacher's paintings are a tribute to the Chassidic way of life and a service to God that spread light in a dark world, enriching our hearts and minds. They connect us to God. She likes to do acts of kindness and service with her art.

If you wish to purchase an original painting or print from this book, please contact Shoshannah Brombacher at *shoshbm@gmail.com.*

CPSIA information can be obtained
at www.ICGtesting.com
Printed in the USA
FSOW01n1245020916
24550FS